SAINTS

FOR THE

SICK

". . . Gladly therefore will I glory in my infirmities, that the power of Christ may dwell in me." —2 Corinthians 12:9

SAINTS
FOR THE
SICK

By

Joan Carroll Cruz

"My grace is sufficient for thee: for power is made perfect in infirmity."
—2 Corinthians 12:9

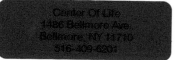

OTHER BOOKS BY THE AUTHOR

Saintly Men of Modern Times   *Secular Saints*
Saintly Women of Modern Times   *The Incorruptibles*
Saintly Children and Teens of Modern Times *Prayers and Heavenly Promises*
Mysteries, Marvels, Miracles   *Eucharistic Miracles*
Miraculous Images of Our Lord   *Relics*
Miraculous Images of Our Lady   *Desires of Thy Heart*

Nihil Obstat: Rev. Terry T. Tekippe
               Censor Librorum

Imprimatur: ✠ Most Rev. Francis B. Schulte
               Archbishop of New Orleans
               October 28, 1998

The Imprimatur is the Church's declaration that a work is free from error in matters of faith and morals and in no way implies that the Church endorses the contents of the manuscript.

ISBN: 978-0-89555-832-9

Printed and bound in the United States of America.

TAN Books
Charlotte, North Carolina
2010

This book is dedicated to the memory of my son,
Michael David Cruz.

CONTENTS

AUTHOR'S NOTE

Our Lord once said, "The poor you have always with you." (*Matthew* 26:11). The same might also be said of the sick, who are all about us, suffering in one way or another from conditions that are annoying, serious, or life-threatening. For the suffering souls who have come to our attention, would it not be comforting and reassuring for them to find a Saint who endured the same problems—one who understands the difficulties and would willingly pray for them? Here you will find scores of Saints and a list of well over 100 physical conditions which these saintly, suffering souls accepted as the will of God. (When referring to those not canonized, we are of course using the term "Saint" in an unofficial sense.)

Counted among them are priests and nuns, nobles and the humble, martyrs, mothers and fathers, teenagers and even children. All bear a title, that of either Saint, Blessed, Venerable or Servant of God, whose causes for beatification have been accepted by the Vatican. Accounts of many of the heroic sufferings of those listed here have been generously provided by those who attended them and by those family members who are anxious to demonstrate the saintly qualities of their relatives. Here you will find saintly persons who suffered atrocious pains, yet they suffered patiently and without complaint, while offering their pains for the salvation of souls and for the good of the Church.

How were these Saints able to accept their sufferings so patiently and with confidence in the mercy of God? They had a secret, and it is this: time after time, it is found that when the sufferers abandoned themselves completely to God's holy will, they were given the grace to accept their sufferings willingly and without complaint.

While reading these biographies, it is to be remembered that not all medical conditions progress in the same manner. What a current patient is enduring will not necessarily worsen, or develop complications, or even be life-threatening, as was the ailment of the Saint who suffered the same sickness. It is to be considered that medical science has vastly improved, with more advanced diagnostic methods, new medications, new procedures and cures. In fact, after reading about the resignation of these holy souls and their determination to accept willingly the plan of God for them, the reader, it is hoped, will feel inclined to invoke these holy souls; as a result, his condition may very well improve. If not, then through the example of these holy souls the reader will surely be given the grace to accept his condition with more patience and confidence in the merciful love of God.

For those who cannot find a Saint whose condition is like their own, it is recommended that they read the chapter about Venerable Mari Carmen Gonzalez-Valerio, who was only nine years old at her death; Venerable Anne de Guigné, who was 11; St. Lydwine of Schiedam, who endured a whole catalog of sufferings; and Bl. Margaret of Castello, who was born hunchbacked, dwarfed, blind and lame. A list at the back of the book gives various physical conditions and the Saints who endured them as recommendations or suggestions of whom to pray to for assistance in various types of ailments.

It is my hope that patients will find here a source of encouragement in their sufferings and perhaps may select one or two of these saintly souls as their advocates in Heaven. Writing this book has been an inspiration to me, as I pray reading it will be an inspiration for you.

Joan Carroll Cruz

SAINTS

FOR THE

SICK

"For as the sufferings of Christ abound in us: so also by Christ doth our comfort abound." —2 Corinthians 1:5

1. Saint Albert the Great
(Albertus Magnus) (c. 1206-1280)

HE WAS called by his contemporaries "The wonder and miracle of our age." Seven centuries later Pope Pius XI still recognized him as a great writer whose works, in addition to those on theology and philosophy, included writings on botany, mineralogy, astronomy, physics, chemistry, anthropology, cosmography and many other subjects. His study of nature included the writing and cataloging of 114 species of birds and of various aquatic animals, serpents and other creatures. He was familiar with medicinal herbal remedies, surgery, medicines and even dentistry. As to philosophy and theology, he had no equal. At the time of his death it was said: "He knew everything that was knowable."

St. Albert was born the eldest son of the Count of Bollstadt in Lauingen, Swabia, Bavaria about the year 1206. We know nothing of his earlier training, but we do know that he studied at the University of Padua and joined the Order of St. Dominic in 1223. His studies continued at various universities. He apparently passed his subjects with great distinction, so that he almost immediately began teaching theology in Hildesheim. Albert then returned to Paris, where he received a Doctor's degree in theology and resumed his teaching career. One of his students in Paris was the great St. Thomas Aquinas, whose genius Albert quickly recognized. St. Albert became the spiritual director of St. Thomas and also predicted his future greatness.

For a time St. Albert served as Provincial of his Order in Germany, and he was also consecrated bishop. He retained the office of Bishop of Regensburg for three years, until his resignation—which was accepted with reluctance. St. Albert then resumed his work at the university and wrote numerous books that are still highly esteemed. Later he retired to various houses of the Order, where he was known for his virtue and love of the Church, but he continued to preach throughout southern Germany. He also preached the Eighth Crusade in Austria. In his later years he fought vigorously in defense of the orthodoxy of his former pupil, St. Thomas Aquinas. Thomas' death in 1274 caused Albert to weep bitterly, saying, "The light of the Church has been extinguished."

St. Albert's own mental sharpness did not continue to the end of his life. This renowned saint who was a scientist, a writer of great works, a distinguished professor and one who was always studying and preaching had to undergo great humiliations and frustrations when his memory and his intellectual powers began to fail. It is thought that this might have been the result of a stroke.

The saint died sitting in a large chair surrounded by members of his Order who were singing the *Salve Regina* at the time of his passing. He had experienced a full life as a preacher, a teacher, an administrator and an arbiter of peace. In his own lifetime he was known as "The Universal Doctor."

Pope Pius XI wrote of St. Albert: "He was a conspicuously great man in his own age and is still great in our day; by his preeminent qualities as teacher and his surpassing skill in so many departments of knowledge, he has won and deserves the special title of 'The Great.'"

2. Venerable Alberto Capellan Zuazo
(1888-1965)

HIS father of eight children was born in Santo Domingo de la Calzada, Spain. As a young boy he liked to serve Holy Mass and claimed to be a poor student, but as a teenager he claimed to excel in one endeavor, and that was dancing with a group of folk dancers. He was a normal teenager, with many friends, and with them he often played little pranks.

At the age of 21, Alberto won out over many rivals and married his childhood sweetheart, Isabel. For a time he was subject to bad moods and was often verbally abusive to his wife. Although his income from farming was satisfactory, he wrote, "I lacked something to be happy. What? Simply, God was with me, but I was not with Him. My heart looked at the earth, but little to the sky. That was the secret."

Almost all we know of Alberto comes from two school notebooks which he started writing in 1943. In them we learn that a change in his soul occurred when a neighbor gave him a copy of the Catechism, which fascinated him. As a result, Alberto became a changed man. He began to attend Holy Mass daily before going into his fields to work, and he gradually developed two great interests: night adoration of the Blessed Sacrament and a love for the poor. Alberto was so devoted to his hour of adoration that he was elected president of the Nocturnal Adoration Society in his area, and then he was re-elected president for 11 consecutive terms.

For the homeless, Alberto offered his barn as a shelter, and he eventually constructed a building that he called the *Recogimiento,* meaning the "Collection" or the "Gathering." He provided beds, blankets and all else that was needed. In the *Recogimiento* the poor felt secure and welcome, and they were assisted by Alberto in countless ways. In addition, he opened his home to shepherd boys during the winter, and at night he taught them the basics of reading, writing, and the first notions of arithmetic. He is known to have been called often to the homes of the poor and to have gone without complaint or hesitation. Testimonials of his aid to the poor and homeless are numerous.

When Alberto reached retirement age, he began to experience angina and chest pains, which he said was the beginning of his Purgatory. Eventually, he experienced a heart attack. He died quietly on February 24, 1965 at the age of 77.

One of Alberto's sons, Gerardo, a missionary priest in Burundi, gave a glowing testimony of his father's life, which includes these words: "In those days, we were given the impression that God was severe, but my father knew that God was merciful, understanding and a friend, and this greatly impressed us. . . . From the time of his conversion he was faithful to his devotions, to the Angelus, to his nocturnal visits to the Blessed Sacrament and to the recitation of the daily Rosary." Based on the entries in Alberto's notebooks, from the time of his conversion he had spent 660 vigils of adoration before the Blessed Sacrament.

The Congregation for the Causes of Saints issued the Decree *Super Virtutibus* in 1998, giving Alberto the title of Venerable.

3. SAINT ALDEGUND (c. 630-684)

ALDEGUND was born in Hainault, France about the year 630, the daughter of Walbert, who was of royal descent. While very young, Aldegund consecrated herself to God by a vow of chastity and resisted all proposals of marriage, remaining in the house of her pious parents until she took the religious veil. She founded and governed a great house of holy virgins at Maubeuge, where she experienced many revelations. For reasons not specified, she was often tried by slanders, crosses and persecutions, for which she begged the mercy of Almighty God.

After a time, she developed a cancer in the breast causing pains which she accepted patiently for the salvation of sinners. In addition to the agony she experienced, she was also afflicted by the ministrations of surgeons who cauterized the wound and made numerous incisions, which only brought about more pain and discomfort.

St. Aldegund is said to have died of her condition in a rapture of ardent love on January 30, 684.

4. SERVANT OF GOD ALDO BLUNDO
(1919-1934)

HIS life is said to have been a "pilgrimage of pain, which was illuminated by his faith and by his great spirit of prayer . . . an unusual spiritual ascension at his tender age, which was fed by the Holy Eucharist."

Aldo was born in Naples, Italy, on January 23, 1919, and was soon inflicted with a variety of ailments. The poor child suffered in infancy with problems that centered around the lungs. Until the age of five, he suffered from pleurisy, bronchitis and pneumonia, which developed into a persistent cough that affected the throat. He had difficulty in moving, which the doctors diagnosed as hypertrophy, an abnormal enlargement of the muscles. In his case, this condition involved the pelvic region and progressed into a paralysis. As if these problems were not enough, Aldo was also diagnosed with eye problems—specifically, progressive degenerate myopia (nearsightedness). Thus at the age of eight, he was found to have failing eyesight and was condemned to immobility. Another tragic condition followed when Aldo fell and broke his leg, which never healed properly.

Now confined to bed or a wheelchair, Aldo was free to move only his head and his hands. For the next few years of his life, he suffered terribly, but he was resigned to his pains because he was inspired by the Passion of Our Lord. He declared one day that he was offering his life for the salvation of sinners. His example of patient suffering and his inspired pronouncements deeply affected his family and all who came into contact with him, especially his father, who was a non-practicing Catholic.

Determined to help his son, Aldo's father, with the best of intentions, had him undergo physical therapy, electrotherapy and drug therapy, as well as other procedures, which only added to the youngster's sufferings, but without a favorable result. Aldo once asked his father, "Why waste so much money? Only the Madonna can help me."

Aldo was taken on a pilgrimage to the shrine of Our Lady of the Rosary in 1929 when he was ten years old, and five years later was brought to Lourdes. His cure was not the Will of God, but Aldo accepted this in good faith, offering his sufferings for wayward youth and for priests.

His constant reply when asked how he felt was: "I am fine, my pains are not so bad." His answer was always given with a smile.

Aldo was particularly devoted to the Rosary, which he prayed with his eyes closed, in deep meditation. He was devoted to the Apostolate of Prayer and wanted his whole family to be consecrated to the Sacred Heart of Jesus. He was especially pleased when he was enrolled in the Association of the Perpetual Rosary.

Having suffered from infancy from various painful infirmities and the pains associated with his paralysis, Aldo died at the age of 15 in Naples on December 5, 1934. Twenty-four years later, in 1958, his cause for beatification was accepted by the Vatican.

5. SERVANT OF GOD
ALEXIA GONZALEZ-BARROS (1971-1985)

ALEXIA had the good fortune to be born into a loving and deeply religious family. Her parents gave their seven children a well-rounded Catholic education. While Alexia participated in all the prayers and devotions of the family, she was still a normal girl who liked nice clothes, attended movies and loved sailing. She was a regular girl in all respects, yet her sanctity in the face of an agonizing illness is now being recognized around the world.

Since Alexia was born several years after the sixth child, she was the darling of the family, but despite the attention and love she received, she never took advantage of it. She was generous with her brothers and sisters, as well as with her classmates when she started school at the age of four. At the age of six, Alexia made her first Confession and frequently recited the Rosary. One day Alexia's mother, after seeing her daughter make two very reverential genuflections before the tabernacle, asked Alexia about her action. Alexia's reply was startling: "I tell Him things, Mommy. I say: 'Jesus, may I always do what You want.'" This phrase would be repeated by Alexia throughout her brief life.

All went well until the spring of 1984, when Alexia was 13. It was then that the healthy-looking girl started speaking of having back pains. Nothing appeared on the x-rays, but when she mentioned that "I can't move my hand," more x-rays followed. It was then that the doctor discovered that Alexia's spinal column was damaged in such a way that if she moved, paralysis would result. Thus began a veritable martyrdom for the young girl.

Alexia's first operation lasted four hours and consisted of implanting a portion of her hip bone into her spinal column to secure a break that had been discovered. To avoid pressure, she was placed in a traction device that kept her spinal column extended. Despite these treatments, she often endured painful arm cramps, and her weak legs gradually become paralyzed. Nevertheless, in spite of all, Alexia's spirits remained high.

Because her condition did not improve, Alexia was then examined by a different set of doctors. They discovered a tumor in the cervical vertebrae that had not been detected earlier and which was pressing on the spinal column. A second operation was necessary to remove the tumor. To prepare for this, Alexia confessed her faults, received Holy Communion and prayed quietly for over half an hour. Later she prayed: "Jesus, I want You to cure me. I want to get well. But if You don't want it that way, then I want to do what You want."

This second operation lasted three hours. Afterward, it was found that the tumor was malignant. Soon after, Alexia mentioned that the incision made during the first operation was hurting badly. Since that incision had never healed, it was now carefully examined. This examination revealed that pieces of gauze had been left in the wound during the first operation.

Eight days after the operation, the diagnosis was made that Alexia had Ewing's Sarcoma, an extremely grave but curable cancer. As part of her treatment, Alexia was given large amounts of medications which produced nausea, vomiting and legs cramps. Then she was fitted with a head-to-shoulder brace. While enduring her pains she was heard to repeatedly pray: "Jesus, may I always do what You want."

Many difficulties arose during Alexia's treatment: a catheter had to be inserted into the jugular vein; punctures with large needles had to be made in her back, causing wounds which promptly festered; and sores appeared in her mouth and throat, making it difficult for her to speak and eat.

Yet another operation was scheduled, this time to correct the first grafting and to destroy any residue from the tumor. On the morning of the operation, Alexia devoutly received Holy Communion and then endured 17 hours in the operating room. After this, she was placed in a partial cast with a metallic crown around her head which was held in place by four screws imbedded in her skull.

Finally, a fourth operation became necessary; it lasted eight hours. Afterward, Alexia still had to wear the cast and the metallic crown, and there were new surgical wounds at the back of her neck and on her hip, both of which refused to heal. The brave little girl endured everything with patience and not a word of complaint—a very surprising situation, since she was enduring oppressive heat, immobility, potent medications, unbearable headaches, chemotherapy, the uncomfortable partial brace, the metallic crown and numerous injections.

It was soon discovered that a condition known as metastasis in the meninges had developed. This was a hopeless condition.

Alexia again accepted her condition with its grim prognosis and continued her customary prayers. Her mother placed a scapular of Our Lady of Mount Carmel around her daughter's neck and placed in her hands a rosary. The hospital chaplain heard her Confession, gave her Holy Communion and administered the Sacraments of Confirmation and Anointing of the Sick, which Alexia received with keen attention. She made frequent spiritual communions, and because of her difficulty in swallowing, she received only small pieces of the Blessed Sacrament.

During her final days, her sanctity was observed by all who

came in contact with her. One doctor exclaimed as he left the room, "This is the anteroom to Heaven." A non-practicing Catholic nurse once remarked, "I can't enter that room. How can one die with so much joy?" Another declared, "She is a child saint." And a priest who often visited announced: "When someone asks me what I saw in Alexia, the only thing that comes to my mind is this: sanctity."

While at the University Hospital in Navarre, Alexia pronounced these reassuring words: "Believe it or not, God sends the strength you need and even makes you smile about it."

Oxygen relieved some of Alexia's difficulties in breathing, but now she was apparently going blind. Despite this, she seemed aware that her guardian angel, whom she had named Hugo, sometimes left her side, but she exclaimed, "I know! We'll go to Heaven together, and when we get there I won't mind if he wants to be with the other angels."

During Alexia's last moments her mother asked her, "Alexia, do you love Jesus?" The answer was a firm, "Yes." Then she was asked, "And are you happy?" Alexia once again answered, "Yes" and breathed her last. It was December 5, 1985.

After her death one of the doctors predicted to the family, "Someday we shall see this child honored on the altars of the Church."

Biographies of Alexia were soon written and spread throughout the world, resulting in countless letters being sent to the family for more information. Prayer cards were printed, while Alexia's prayer, "May I always do what You want," was adopted by many.

Documents are now being prepared for the introduction of a cause for beatification.

6. BLESSED ALPAIS (d. 1211)

ORN into a poor peasant family at Cudot in the diocese of Orleans, France, Alpais became bedridden with leprosy while still very young. As a result of the disease, she first lost the use of her arms, and then of her legs. Known for her holiness and mortifications, Alpais also became well known for the gift of inedia, by which she subsisted solely on the Holy Eucharist. To verify this condition, a commission was appointed by the Holy See, which examined and confirmed the truth of this holy fast. Out of reverence for her condition, those who loved her built a church next to her hovel with a special window, from which she could conveniently attend services and the Holy Sacrifice of the Mass.

Because of the many miracles worked by this fervent soul, as well as her ecstatic states, Alpais' little dwelling became a place of pilgrimage, with prelates and nobles coming from all parts to see and consult with her. Queen Adela, wife of Louis VII of France, visited Alpais on several occasions.

Her cultus, which began right from the time of her death in 1211, was confirmed by Bl. Pope Pius IX in 1874. A biography of this saintly woman was written by a contemporary while Blessed Alpais was still living.

7. SERVANT OF GOD ALPHONSUS LAMBE
(1932-1959)

ALFIE, as he was called, was blessed to be part of a genuinely Christian family, whose piety drew him to all things religious. He was born at Tullamore, Ireland, and at the age of 13 he declared his intention to become a Christian Brother. He was received with others into the novitiate and became an ideal novice, diligent in his studies, active in games, and devout in his prayers.

But Alfie was given to fainting spells. The doctor who examined him declared that he would never be able to endure the rigors of religious life. The superior of the community advised that he return home and come back when he was better. This was a great disappointment for Alfie. Instead of working for God in the religious life, he now had to take up employment as an office worker in the secular world.

Since he felt the need to work for God, Alfie joined the Legion of Mary in Tullamore. At 18 years of age, therefore, he plunged wholeheartedly into making home and hospital visitations, serving the parish and ministering to gypsies, who often passed through Tullamore.

When the mill for which he was working closed, Alfie saw a providential opportunity and offered all his time and energies to the Legion. Alfie and another Legion member named Seamus Grace were accepted as envoys and were sent to Venezuela, South America.

After a time Seamus Grace was hospitalized, so that Alfie had to work alone for a time, that is, until those he had attracted to the Legion began to help him in his work. He became so well known in Venezuela that he was gradually invited to introduce the Legion of Mary into Ecuador, Brazil, Colombia, Bolivia, Chile, Paraguay, Uruguay and Argentina.

Alfie's charm, persistence, persuasive talents, and hard work attracted many to the Legion. In fact, a senator, a school teacher, and a judge on the Supreme Court of Venezuela began helping in the charities of the Legion.

Alfie saw to it that the Legion of Mary was established not only in parishes, but also in leper communities and in prisons. The conversions and attendance at Masses soon became overwhelming.

Bishops were pleased with the success of the Legion. Eventually, newspapers became interested, and regular time slots on the radio were given to the Legion for news of its activities and for the recitation of the Rosary and other prayers.

Unfortunately, Alfie was growing very weak, due in part to dysentery. He often fainted, but he would resume his work once he had gathered enough strength. As his health deteriorated, Alfie's blood pressure fell alarmingly, and he showed signs of nervous exhaustion. He developed severe pains in his stomach, which produced numerous episodes of vomiting blood. Tests revealed the problem to be a bleeding ulcer. Surgery to correct the condition revealed not only the stomach ulcer but also lymphosarkoma, an aggressive malignant tumor. All of Alfie's organs were affected. His condition was declared hopeless.

Alfie suffered through most of January and was finally administered the Last Sacraments by Cardinal Copello. He died on January 21, 1959 at the age of 26.

After his mother decided that Alfie's body should not be returned home, but instead should rest in the country of his spiritual conquests, a large crowd, including bishops, accompanied his body to the grave.

One of the Christian Brothers of Buenos Aires wrote: "The underlying quality of his personality was surely his ardent thirst for souls. It ruled every action of his life. Fed and nourished and encouraged at the banquet table of the Lamb, urged on to ever greater efforts under the over-shadowing mantle of his Blessed Mother, he considered no obstacle too great, no hardship too severe, if by overcoming those handicaps he could win just one soul for Christ."

Alfie's cause for beatification was introduced on June 17, 1987.

8. SAINT ALPHONSUS LIGUORI
(1696-1787)

ALPHONSUS Liguori was the first of the seven children born in Marianella, near Naples, to a family that belonged to the Neapolitan nobility. At an early age he showed an extraordinary aptitude for study, and he entered law school at the age of 16. After receiving degrees in both civil and canon law, he began to practice his chosen profession at the amazing age of 18. It is reported that during the several years that he practiced law, he never lost a case. But then, after losing an important case due to an oversight, he abandoned his legal career and, despite his father's opposition, entered the seminary in preparation for the priesthood.

Ordained at the age of 30, St. Alphonsus was assigned first to an apostolate for the homeless and marginalized youth of Naples. For these he founded "Evening Chapels" where the youngsters found schooling, prayer and social activities. At the time of the saint's death, there were 72 of these chapels in existence, with more than 10,000 active participants.

It was soon realized that the scope of the work, which also included the elderly, required additional help. Fr. Alphonsus then founded the Congregation of the Most Holy Redeemer, known as the Redemptorists, whose goals were to teach and preach in the slums. Later, the Redemptorists' zeal for souls extended to the care of the sick. The new order was established when the young priest was only 36 years old. It consisted, in the beginning, of only three other priests. Shortly afterward, a companion order of nuns was founded by Sister Maria Celeste.

Through the long years of his life, Alphonsus administered the Congregation's affairs and also found time to write, teach and give spiritual advice.

When Alphonsus was 62 years old, despite being ill, he was notified that he had been chosen bishop of the diocese of Sant'Agata dei Goti. Declaring himself unfit to properly care for the people who would be placed under his care, he wrote to Pope Clement XIII asking to be excused because of age and health. At the time, the saint was asthmatic, lame, bent over, partly blind and partially deaf. But the Pope insisted, and Alphonsus was consecrated in April of 1762.

During his years in the bishopric of Sant'Agata dei Goti, Alphonsus became so ill that he received the Last Sacraments four times. Ten years later he again pleaded to be relieved of his office, listing his various ailments in a letter to Pope Pius VI. The saint wrote: "I am in extreme old age, for in the month of September I enter on my eightieth year. I have many infirmities which warn me that death is near. I suffer from a weakness of the chest which several times has reduced me to the last extremity, and from palpitations of the heart. . . . At present I am suffering from such constant headaches that sometimes they make me like one deprived of his faculties. Besides these evils, I am subject to various dangerous attacks which I have to remedy by blood-letting, blisters and other remedies."

As if that were not enough, the saint added: "My hearing fails me so that it is difficult to hear Confessions. I am paralyzed to such an extent that I can no longer write a line. With difficulty I sign my name. . . . I am become so crippled that I can no longer walk a step and have need of two assistants to help me. I pass my time on a bed or alone in a chair . . ."

It is interesting to note that St. Alphonsus' assistants contrived a chair—which they called a "roller chair"—with which he was moved from one place to another. This was a great convenience, but the saint constantly worried that the noise of the chair disturbed others at prayer.

The crippled condition that St. Alphonsus described is believed to have been rheumatoid arthritis. Additionally, in extreme old age the saint's head was abnormally bent forward to such an extent that his chin rested on his chest, causing a furious sore. This is the reason his portraits usually depict him with his head bent forward.

Finally, in 1775, Pope Pius VI released him from his duties. St. Alphonsus was 79 and had served as bishop for 13 years.

Somehow over the years he succeeded, despite his many infirmities, in writing 111 books of spirituality and theology, of which *The Glories of Mary* is said to be the most widely read book on the Blessed Virgin in the world. With good reason St. Alphonsus is regarded as the most prolific writer in the history of the Church. The saint was also multi-talented in that he played the piano and wrote 50 hymns, some of which can still be found in various hymnals.

St. Alphonsus Liguori died on August 1, 1787 at the age of 91, surrounded by members of his community. He was canonized in 1831 by Pope Gregory XVI and was proclaimed a Doctor of the Church in 1871. In 1950 he was declared Patron of Confessors and Moralists.

9. BLESSED AMADEUS IX (1435-1472)

AMADEUS was the privileged son of Duke Louis I of Savoy (now southeastern France) and Anne of Cyprus. While still an infant, Amadeus was betrothed to Yolande, daughter of Charles VII of France. It was hoped that this union would bring peace between Savoy and France. The marriage took place when Amadeus was 16. The union proved to be a happy one, but of the couple's four sons and two daughters, most died at an early age.

Amadeus was handsome, accomplished and endowed with exceptional graces, but unfortunately he was subject all his life to severe attacks of epilepsy, which at times completely prostrated and incapacitated him. After these attacks he would remark to his worried attendants, "Why concern yourselves? Humiliations give access to the Kingdom of God."

In spite of this condition, Amadeus was extremely austere in his private life and never excused himself because of his delicate health. He began each day with private meditation and the Holy Mass, and he received the Sacraments more frequently than was customary.

Amadeus lived happily with his wife and children in the Province of Brescia, which had been given to him as his portion. However, when his father died, he was called upon to govern Savoy and Piedmont (now northwestern Italy). During his seven-year reign, he was successful in reducing bribery and in preventing the oppression of the poor by the rich. He could not bring himself to refuse alms to anyone, and he is known to have frequently exhausted the contents of his purse. He once removed his jeweled collar, broke it into pieces, and distributed the fragments.

Through his wise administration, Amadeus was able to pay the debts of his predecessors, and instead of his many charities being a strain on the treasury, through the grace of God the amount in the treasury was actually increased.

Amadeus was known for having a forgiving nature. He bore malice to no one, including his brothers, who rebelled against him on more than one occasion.

When his epileptic seizures became more numerous and burdensome, Amadeus consigned the government to the hands of his wife. When his subjects rose in revolt on another occasion, Amadeus was imprisoned, but he was freed by King Louis XI of France, who was his brother-in-law. Only a few years later, after receiving the Sacraments, Amadeus died at the age of 37 years. His last words were given to his children: "Be just, love the poor, and the Lord will give peace to your lands." Amadeus was greatly admired and loved by his subjects and was deeply mourned.

10. SERVANT OF GOD AMATA CERRETELLI
(1907-1963)

MATA was not only sickly from the day of her birth, she also suffered from a variety of illnesses during her 56 years. She was born in Campi Besenzio (a village outside Florence, Italy) and was so frail at her birth that she was baptized the same day. For the next nine years, she suffered from what the doctors diagnosed as rheumatism. She could walk only with great difficulty, and in a stooped posture. These conditions continued, and then, at age 18, she also developed a speech defect. Later, her health declined still further, with the diagnosis being infected tonsils. An operation for their removal was performed, but because of her frail condition, the procedure was done without anesthesia. Amata did not improve, so the doctor amended his diagnosis to include trouble with her kidneys and spine. Once again she was bedridden, this time with a tumor on the bottom of her foot. An operation to remove it was performed in the doctor's office, but the tumor returned. No sooner was this last problem taken care of than Amata developed further problems—this time with her throat, which required another operation. As a result, Amata experienced slurred speech for the rest of her life.

Amata eventually found work in a shop that manufactured artificial flowers and decorative feathers. She worked at this occupation for two years in spite of suffering from a variety of illnesses. First, two abscesses developed around her nose that caused a swelling of her whole head and an inability to eat or drink. Then a high fever confined her to bed. After this, she suffered a sciatica attack in her left thigh. When this subsided, a soreness in a finger of her left hand caused such pain that a doctor recognized it as an infection under the nail and removed it, again without an anesthetic. A second nail was also removed. Next, Amata's appendix was removed, as was a large quantity of infectious material from her abdomen.

When World War II started, Amata twice escaped injury when bombs exploded near her. Despite all the privations brought about by the War, she helped those who were worse off than herself. She is noted for having cared for an elderly, paralyzed niece of the parish priest, continuing to do so until the woman's death. During this time she also cared for her widowed mother, who was ill from a lack of nourishment. But again Amata herself fell ill, this time with a condition that provoked vomiting, which completely baffled the doctors. A cyst then developed on her left eyelid, requiring an operation to correct the eye, which had been rendered immobile. Next, she was diagnosed with tuberculosis.

When the tuberculosis was under control, Amata and a friend asked to be accepted as tertiaries in the Order of the Carmelites of the Ancient Observance. Father Augustine Bartolini became Amata's spiritual adviser in 1948 and helped her to form the apostolate known as "The Family," which developed into several branches, each working in a different area of need. Suffering physically and financially all her life, Amata continued to help others who were in need, and through her organization she assisted countless fellow sufferers. Helped through The Family were victims of prejudice, dishonesty or cruel poverty, as well as those ostracized by society, including adulterers and even lepers.

Amata was already well advanced in the spiritual life because of her acceptance of suffering as the Will of God, and under

Father Augustine's guidance, she progressed even more rapidly. She was especially devoted to the Blessed Sacrament and spent hours in deep contemplation. She was also devoted to the souls in Purgatory, and she accepted her sufferings and made other sacrifices for their relief. Toward the end of her life, Amata exclaimed, "I'm no longer good for anything. I only know how to suffer!"

In January of 1963, Amata developed a severe cold that became progressively worse, with a high fever and spasms that shook her whole body. She received the Sacrament of the Anointing of the Sick—which was then called Extreme Unction or Last Anointing—and remained conscious for some time before falling into a coma. Amata died on January 26, 1963 in the presence of members of The Family.

At the time of Amata's death, there were several thousand members in The Family, which continues to this day to bring charity to those in need.

11. SERVANT OF GOD ANFROSINA BERARDI
(1920-1933)

ANFROSINA was born into a modest farming family in San Marco di Preturo, Italy on December 6, 1920. From early childhood she was known for her practice of virtue and for her gentle nature, especially when troubles arose among the siblings of the large family of nine children.

When Anfrosina was only 11 years old she was suddenly stricken with an attack of appendicitis. Her family thought she might improve, but when she grew worse, she was taken to the hospital at Aquila. She endured excruciating pains for four days before undergoing an operation, which proved to be unsuccessful. Infection began and spread throughout her abdomen, producing spasmodic cramps. It was the heroic acceptance of these acute pains that showed Anfrosina's extraordinary virtue, which became known throughout the area.

When the townspeople learned that she was accepting her painful condition without complaint for the love of God, they and many others from nearby areas paid visits to her bedside. Many reformed their lives, while others were inspired to a life of prayer. Almost all petitioned her to pray for them and their intentions. In spite of her visitors being very numerous, Anfrosina greeted everyone with a smile and a word of welcome.

When her mother seemed especially worried about her daughter's condition, Anfrosina reminded her that the Blessed Virgin was looking after her, and that after she died, her mother should not cry because it would be a happy event. After all, she was going to meet the Madonna.

The brave little girl suffered acutely for two years before dying piously on March 13, 1933. She was so highly regarded that she was buried, not in the local cemetery, but in the parish church of St. Mark at Preturo, the city of her birth, in the church where she had so often received the Sacraments.

Devotees are still attracted to this saintly young girl, so much so that the Archbishop of Aquila has begun the informative process for the cause for her beatification.

12. Servant of God Angela Iacobellis
(1948-1961)

NGELA was born in Rome on October 16, 1948 and was given the privilege of being baptized in St. Peter's Basilica. Because of the difficulties of the postwar years, the family moved to Naples, where Angela would spend the rest of her life. She had many talents and was such a good student that she was often assigned to help slower students with their schoolwork. She loved listening to music, dancing, and above all, sketching, having made many amusing caricatures of people she loved.

When Angela was only 12 years old, tragedy struck. After she suddenly lost her appetite and became very pale and weak, her mother took her for tests—which revealed that Angela had leukemia. She knew nothing of the grim results of the tests until she was taken on a pilgrimage to Lourdes, where relatives pleaded for a miracle. Angela accepted calmly the news of her condition, and she told her mother not to worry, for she had asked the help of the Madonna of the Rosary, whose magnificent shrine was located in Pompeii, not far from Naples.

For a time Angela was well enough to attend school—that is, until she experienced a hemorrhage from the nose. Numerous blood transfusions were ordered, all without favorable results. Angela became so weak that at Christmas time she lost all interest in her presents and found comfort only in her Rosary, which she recited frequently. She derived additional comfort from holding close to her heart the relics of St. Thérèse and Pope St. Pius X.

All who attended Angela during her illness, as well as all her visitors, were edified by her acceptance of her situation as the Will of God and by her willingness to suffer for souls without complaint.

After suffering a respiratory crisis on March 27, 1961, Angela died—but with such a pleasant expression on her face that relatives did not suspect that she was dead.

Burial first took place in the Church of St. Clare in Naples, where she had asked to be buried, but later her body was transferred to a chapel dedicated to her in the Church of St. Giovanni dei Fiorentini. At that time, November 21, 1997, a canonical recognition was made for the cause of her beatification. To everyone's astonishment, the body was found to be perfectly preserved after 36 years.

News of the pious 13-year-old girl and her willingness to accept her painful condition for the love of God spread beyond Italy, with many favorable answers to prayer resulting from her intercession.

13. Servant of God Angelina Pirini
(1922-1940)

NGELINA was born in northeastern Italy to a prayerful family. She excelled in her school work but remained in school only until the fifth grade. As a means of helping with the financial condition of the family, she was apprenticed to a tailor. When not at work in the tailor shop, she was at home helping her mother with the household chores, which she performed responsibly and generously. At the age of 12, Angelina felt the need to assist at Mass every day. She progressed rapidly in prayer, once writing, "O Jesus, You are my only love—my thoughts are always fixed on You. . . . I feel that the divine love has completely invaded my spirit, and I feel myself burn from this inextinguishable flame." This love of God prompted Angelina to join an organization known as Catholic Action, which participated in various charitable activities.

Her advance in the spiritual life was duly noted by her spiritual director, Fr. Joseph Marchi, who gave her permission to make a temporary vow of virginity at the age of 15. She made a perpetual vow a year later.

Soon after making her perpetual vow, Angelina was stricken with appendicitis. She underwent an operation, but it was unsuccessful. A second operation revealed an incurable intestinal tuberculosis. The pains she suffered she offered in reparation for the sins of the world and in particular for the sanctification of priests. She accepted all her sufferings with great serenity and interior joy, which edified all who came into contact with her.

A year later, on June 16, 1938, the Feast of Corpus Christi, Angelina consecrated herself in a special way to the Holy Will of God. She died four months afterwards, on October 2, 1940, being only 18 years old.

We learn of Angelina's intense spiritual life, her love of God and the Blessed Virgin from her diary, which she entitled "Spiritual Accounts and the Spiritual Will." Angelina's bravery during her time of intense pain prompted the local bishop to open the cause for her beatification.

14. Servant of God Angiolino Bonetta
(1948-1963)

NGIOLINO was born in northern Italy to a truck-driving father and a mother who worked as a cloth repairer. During his early years he was affectionate, athletic, and was described as being playful and mischievous, but good and generous with everyone.

After receiving his First Holy Communion, Angiolino seems to have changed and to have concentrated more on the practice of virtue, although he still excelled scholastically and athletically, participating in races, football and other athletic endeavors. When his right knee began to trouble him, this was blamed on his activities and on the occasional falls he suffered during his activities. However, when he began to lose weight and began limping, his mother took him to the hospital for radiological examinations. The tests revealed bone cancer. Angiolino was then only 12 years old.

The young boy abandoned himself to the Will of God and willingly endured chemotherapy treatments, and then later, the amputation of his leg. To a nun who suggested that he offer his sufferings for souls, he responded, "I have already offered all to Jesus for the conversion of sinners. I am not afraid; Jesus always comes to help me." It is known that Angiolino's cheerful acceptance of his condition obtained several conversions.

Unfortunately, the cancer metastasized, causing extreme pain. Medical procedures added to the distress, but Angiolino prayed to his beloved Madonna, and he was daily supported by his reception of the Holy Eucharist. He was also comforted by holding a crucifix and various other sacramentals that had been given to him, including a relic of St. Bernadette.

The nursing nuns were so edified by their young patient's willing acceptance of pain that they recommended to him certain other patients who were undergoing particularly severe physical or mental suffering. Angiolino is known to have spent many nights praying for these souls by reciting the Holy Rosary, his favorite devotion.

Angiolino was often found absorbed in silent prayer, his eyes closed and a serene expression on his face. The day before he died, in an attempt to console his mother, he told her, "I have made a pact with the Madonna. When the hour arrives, she will come to take me. I have asked her to permit me to make my Purgatory on this earth, not in the other world. When I die, I will immediately fly to Heaven."

Angiolino's death in the early morning hours of January 28, 1963 was truly edifying. While holding his crucifix and relic of St. Bernadette, he looked toward the statue of the Madonna and passed into the next world.

In acknowledgment that Angiolino had reached "breathtaking heights of Christian heroism," his cause for beatification was opened in 1998. This action gave him the title of Servant of God.

15. VENERABLE ANITA CANTIERI
(1910-1942)

ANITA was one of the 12 children born to David Cantieri and Annunziata (Fanucchi) Cantieri. She was born on March 30, 1910 in Lucca, Italy, a city famous as the birthplace of St. Gemma Galgani.

Anita was a healthy and vivacious child, normal in all respects, who knew how to get her way with her siblings. She began attending school at the age of six, and at the age of 13 she transferred to a school operated by the Dorothean nuns, also called the Sisters of St. Dorothy. One of her teachers wrote that Anita was "an example of so many beautiful virtues. She was docile and obedient to the teachers. She was gentle, charitable, silent, helpful to her slow companions, and was often seen in prayer." In fact, Anita attended Mass every day and was often found by her companions in church, where she spent much time in adoration before the tabernacle.

After attending a course of lectures given in 1929 by Father Anzuini of the Company of Jesus, Anita and her companions began working for the Apostolate of Prayer, a work promoted by Father Anzuini. He was to say of her, "This is not a common soul . . . but already very advanced in spirit."

Anita loved the missions. She made clothes for the non-Christian children there. She was also concerned for the poor who were embarrassed that they had no offering to give the priest after Baptisms. She collected money for this purpose and gave what she had collected to a nun, who reported, "Anita would come to me and quietly give me a small sum of money. All her works of charity were performed with so much delicacy and humility that her charity passed unnoticed."

As Anita grew older, her contact with the Sisters of St. Dorothy reinforced her desire for religious life. Her parents objected, but changed their minds after consultations with her confessor. As to the choice of a religious Order, Anita left this entirely to her confessor, Msgr. Angelo Pasquinelli. After he consulted with other priests who knew Anita, it was decided that Anita seemed contemplative and therefore best suited to the life of a Carmelite nun. The order chosen was the Institute of the Tertiary Carmelite Nuns. When a friend of Anita was later puzzling over the choice of a religious Order for herself, Anita told her, "You go to Msgr. Pasquinelli and say to him, 'Monsignor, where does Jesus want me to go?' And then you obey as if God has spoken to you. I did this and my worry was over. I am happy, as I am today."

Anita happily entered the Order, but after a time she developed stomach problems and intermittent fevers, which were diagnosed as an intestinal disorder. When her condition did not improve, she was sent home after 15 months of religious life—but she was encouraged to return when her health improved.

After Anita's return home, the trouble that afflicted her intestines and peritoneum continued. When the doctors seemed grim during their consultations, Anita resigned herself to a life of suffering. Yet she frequently repeated the words, *Deo Gratias*—"Thanks be to God."

Since she knew she would never be well enough to re-enter the convent, nothing prevented her from entering the Third Order Discalced Carmelites (lay Carmelites). She was professed in the Order on July 1, 1935 and was faithful to the observance of the Rule. She read the works of the Carmelite Saints and once wrote: "I love Carmel with a pressing love, but more than that, I love my Lord's will."

Anita also was enrolled in Catholic Action, and when she was able, she was happy to prepare children for their First Holy Communion. She was known in the organization as being a vivacious and happy person "who brightened the weary acts of charity performed by herself and others."

Once again, Anita's physical condition worsened. Peritonitis and fevers were to keep her in bed for the next eight years of her life. She was cared for by her mother and two sisters, from whom she frequently begged pardon for all the trouble she was causing them. Anita never complained, and she always managed a smile, even though she was suffering intensely.

Her spiritual director, Msgr. Pasquinelli, visited her often. To him Anita revealed that she knew the exact day and hour of her death.

In addition to accepting her sufferings from illness, Anita practiced other penances. One penance was to eat without complaint the meals she did not particularly care for. Also, she delayed alleviating her thirst during hot summer months. She even wore instruments of penance, but she never spoke of her sufferings, except when ordered to under obedience.

According to her spiritual director, Anita started receiving people requesting her prayers or seeking comfort in their trials. Soon there was "a constant coming and going." Many told of physical ailments that were small compared to the sufferings endured by Anita, yet in spite of her pains, Anita smiled and continued to offer consolation to those wearied by the trouble of the world.

Anita was now undergoing almost continuous vomiting caused by a tumor that had reached the stomach. She was also afflicted by a tumor in a "delicate part of the body." An operation to remove this problem was performed without an anesthetic. Afterwards, the doctor reported: "In the whole time, not a complaint nor a disorderly gesture was noticed."

Next, Anita's heart became affected with continuous palpitations. She offered these to God, saying, "Dear Lord, every pulsation of my heart is a throb of love for You." The tumor now extended itself from the bowel to the stomach and into the trachea. A surgical intervention was necessary, to which Anita obediently submitted.

Finally, Anita had to endure yet two new ailments: rheumatism and a difficulty with her lungs, in addition to the peritonitis that continued to trouble her intestines. She was to write to a priest, "I resort to obedience and then I am soothed . . . Jesus is so good to me in letting me participate in the sufferings of the cross."

After eight years of what has been described as a "slow and lingering martyrdom," Anita received the Last Sacraments and died on August 24, 1942, the very day she had predicted years earlier.

As soon as her death was announced, those who had visited Anita earlier now returned to report graces received, encouragement in trials, and the return of many to the Sacraments. One priest announced that "a flower has appeared on the earth," while many were applying for relics and for permission to pray in her room.

Anita's cause for beatification was introduced in 1977. She was declared Venerable in 1991.

16. SAINT ANNA ALPHONSA MUTTATHUPADATHU (1910-1946)

ORN in a rural area of Kudamalloor, Kerala, India, Anna lost her mother while very young and was raised by a maternal aunt. At the age of three she contracted a painful eczema, from which she suffered for over a year. Hardly recovered from that, she accidentally fell into a pit of blazing chaff and burned her feet so badly that she was left permanently crippled. In spite of her disability, she was accepted into the Poor Clare Order at Bharananganam in 1928, taking the name Alphonsa. She made her final profession on August 12, 1936.

Alphonsa was assigned to teaching primary grade classes, but she was often absent from the classroom, due to various ailments. These were miraculously cured in November of 1936 through the intervention of Saint Therese of Lisieux and Blessed Kuriakose Elias Chavara. Three years later she suffered from pneumonia, and then, the following year, she experienced a loss of memory that endured for months, due to the shock of having a thief enter her cell. Still suffering weakness as a result of the pneumonia, she was given the Last Rites on September 29, 1941. She promptly regained her memory, although not her health. A few years later, Alphonsa suffered from a stomach problem that began in July of 1945. She endured this for a year before she died of the condition on July 28, 1946.

Throughout her physical trials, Alphonsa was known to have

suffered in silence, to the admiration of her companions in the convent.

Alphonsa was buried in the chapel connected with the cemetery of Saint Mary's church in Bharananganam, India, which has become a place of pilgrimage.

Alphonsa was beatified on February 8, 1986 by Pope John Paul II and canonized on October 12, 2008 by Pope Benedict XVI. She is the first woman from India to be raised to the honors of the altar.

17. SAINT ANNA WANG (1886-1900)

WHEN China was intent on ridding the country of Westerners and Chinese Christians during the Boxer Rebellion of 1900, China made it known that "The government has banned the practice of Western religions. If you renounce your religion, you will be set free; if you refuse, we will kill you." This was said to Anna Wang, whose stepmother had renounced the Faith and had urged Anna to do the same.

Anna refused to submit to the threat by stating: "I believe in God. I am a Christian. I do not renounce God. Jesus save me!"

Anna was to witness the killing of many mothers and their children, even a number of infants. Her response was to kneel in fervent prayer before the carnage. With one of the Boxers standing over her, she was again given the choice of death or the rejection of the Catholic Faith. Anna steadfastly refused, saying, "I prefer to die rather than give up my Faith."

Enraged by her response, the soldier hacked off her right arm and asked her again, "Do you deny your religion?" In spite of her pain, Anna remained silent. She was struck again and then was promptly decapitated. Before the final blow, she was heard to say: "The door of Heaven is open" and to whisper the name of Jesus three times.

The heroic nature of Anna's ordeal is to be admired. This 14-year-old girl bravely reaffirmed her Catholic Faith while she was enduring unspeakable pain and was being covered with blood.

Of all the martyrs of the Boxer rebellion, Anna Wang seems to be the best known. Together with 120 other Christian martyrs, she was canonized by Pope John Paul II on October 1, 2000.

18. Venerable Anne de Guigne
(1911-1922)

ANNE de Guigne, child of a privileged family, was born in the Chateau de la Cour that overlooked the Lake of Annecy, France. She was the first of four children. No one would have predicted that this child would reach the heights of sanctity since she had a tempestuous spirit and was inclined to be bossy with her siblings and older playmates.

After Anne's father, Jacques de Guigne, rejoined his old regiment during World War I, he was wounded on three separate occasions. During his hospitalization for a wound suffered during his third battle, Madame de Guigne permitted Anne to accompany her to the hospital. After seeing the suffering men, including her own father, who was to die soon after, the five-year-old Anne was changed forever.

It was then that she realized that life is fleeting, that sorrows and sufferings frequently occur on earth, and that Heaven was the only place for the good and virtuous. Anne decided upon Heaven, and from then on she became a docile child, obedient to her mother and kind to all she met.

A year later Anne expressed the desire to receive her First Holy Communion, although she was not the proper age. Nevertheless, she was enrolled in catechism class. Her teacher, Mother St. Raymond, wrote that Anne was a very gifted child and not only got along well with her fellow students, but was greatly admired by them. The teacher wrote: "I do not think I ever saw her in a bad humor or upset over anything . . . she never even teased the other children, and this must have meant considerable self-control, for she was naturally so quick and sharp."

Anne had difficulty in memorizing the catechism lessons, but she could explain the answers in clear and precise words. When the teacher asked permission from the Bishop for Anne's early reception of First Holy Communion, the Bishop assigned the superior of the Jesuits to question her. At first the priest scoffed that this tiny girl was old enough; but after hearing Anne's explanations to his questions, he pronounced her ready, remarking to the teacher, "I wish you and I were as well prepared to receive Our Lord as this little girl is."

After receiving the Blessed Sacrament, witnesses remarked that Anne looked positively radiant. On another occasion, when a witness saw the little girl leave the confessional, she exclaimed that Anne seemed absolutely transfigured.

At the time of her First Holy Communion, Anne took as her motto, "Obedience is the sanctity of children." Anne's governess once remarked, "I have never known Anne to refuse a sacrifice." This was said when Anne contracted influenza, and mustard poultices had to be applied to her chest. Even though Anne had to struggle interiorly, she endured all with admirable patience, saying all the time, "Jesus, I offer it to You."

During another illness (para-typhoid) she was required to stay in bed for months and to eat only bland soups for her meals. Once again she made the sacrifice of enduring these tasteless soups without complaint.

Later she was known to have given her sweets and desserts to her siblings and to have played games with them which she did not like. If they wanted her toys, she gladly relinquished them, saying, "'Yes' is the nicest word we can say to Jesus."

Anne was particularly concerned for the poor. Although she

could have asked her wealthy mother for funds to give to the poor, she learned to knit and herself made scarves and other little things to keep them warm.

Anne was ten years old when she gave this wise counsel: "My soul is meant for Heaven. We take a lot of trouble over dressing our bodies, but think less about our souls. . . . There ought to be, first, cleanness (of soul), which means avoiding sin; second, proper clothing, that is, doing our duty; third, adornment, which means the good actions that we do of our own free will. . . . It depends on me. Mother cannot do the work for me."

When Anne was ten years old, she seems to have had a presentiment of her own death. She began speaking of Heaven and seemed eager for the day when she would arrive there. She once told her mother, "I tell Jesus that I love Him . . . I ask Him lots of things, and I pray for sinners too . . . And I tell Him that I want to see Him."

When Anne began to suffer from headaches, she commented, "We have lots of joys here on earth, but they do not last; the only joy that lasts is to have made a sacrifice for Jesus." Eventually the headaches became so severe that Anne found it necessary to remain in bed. Three days later, when the doctor examined her, his diagnosis was meningitis; he did not expect a recovery. Two days later Anne received the Last Anointing, knowing fully what it was. Soon her chest muscles became paralyzed. This caused difficulty in breathing and painful attacks of suffocation that lasted for hours. Through it all, while Anne struggled for breath, she did so without a sign of impatience. Once when her mother told her that her suffering was saving many souls for God, Anne replied with a smile, "Oh, Mother, I'm so glad. If it does that, I will bear lots more."

Anne lingered in pain for some time. Then on January 14, she looked toward a picture of the Blessed Mother and repeated word for word the *Hail Holy Queen*. Then looking at her earthly mother, she died.

Days later, Anne's body was interred in the family vault at Annecy-le-Vieux. In the following years, so many cures and favors were received through her intercession that the Bishop opened the canonical investigation into her life and virtues. The Church's official exhumation and examination of Anne's remains found that her body was perfectly preserved. A declaration of the heroic nature of Anne's virtues was approved by Pope John Paul II on March 3, 1990, giving this almost 11-year-old child the title of Venerable.

19. Servant of God Annie Zelikova
(1924-1941)

THIS simple farm girl had what she called "an apostolate of the smile." She was devoted to St. Thérèse of Lisieux and did well in imitating her virtues. What we know of these efforts is detailed in her record of spiritual exercises, notes from retreats, and letters she wrote as an apostolate.

Annie was born on July 19, 1924 in Moravia, in what is now the Czech Republic. Like most children, she was sometimes headstrong and often wanted her way—that is, until she received her First Holy Communion. From then on she was determined to follow the way of perfection. She attended Holy Mass every day and willingly helped in her father's fields after school. She also kept a little book in which she recorded her thoughts and aspirations and wrote of her love for God.

After attending a retreat, Annie wrote in her little book: "My love was anxious to surrender everything, just so I could be closer to Jesus. My desire began to fly to the very heights of Carmel, in which I perceived that highest union with Jesus. I don't know why I yearned for Carmel right from my childhood years, especially since I never knew a Carmelite. I just knew the Carmelite Little Thérèse; I loved her, and I wanted to imitate her virtuous life . . . I did everything with Jesus. I ran to Him with everything, even with the most ordinary things."

When Annie began to lose weight and to develop a pallid complexion, she was taken to the doctor for X-rays. The diagnosis was not good: advanced tuberculosis. The doctor predicted that Annie would live no more than three months, but she was to live four more years. These would be years spent in great pain, offering everything to God with great love. Annie was pleased that she would be imitating her patroness, St. Thérèse, who had also been stricken with tuberculosis. Because her parents were so worried about her, Annie attempted to relieve their anxiety by attending school and continuing to perform her tasks at home and in the fields. But when she began to cough up blood more frequently, her parents kept her home from school, although she continued to be useful around the house.

When she was 15 she wrote, "Dear Jesus, let my love for You be ever greater, and let that love make me forget myself completely. Everything, whether sorrow or joy, comes from Your love. May everything that I am sing You a song of praise."

Another time she was to write, "How beautiful it is to strive after a strong love which would look only to give honor and glory to Jesus in everything. Every instant it is possible to give Him much . . . All of one's work, every movement, every word can be uttered with great love. Let us do as much as we can, and when we are unsuccessful in something, let us remain peaceful. It depends not so much on the fruit of our work and effort, but rather on the love which led us to that task."

Annie's heart seems to have soared with love when she wrote: "When I'm in the woods or in the garden or even before the tabernacle, I call on every blade of grass, on every flower, on every grain of wheat to praise God. I wish I had as many hearts as there are songs of birds, as there are brooks and springs, as many as there are grains, leaves, as many as there are stars and clouds in heaven, so that I could give enough thanks for the gifts of God."

Annie made another retreat during February of 1940. At that time she recorded thoughts that are reminiscent of St. Thérèse:

"I found true beauty, which is hidden in faithfulness in little things. I always desired to do great and heroic deeds of love, but when I saw that I was unable, I was grieved by it. Now I find great heroism precisely in little things, so that now I haven't the slightest regret whether I can do something or not."

Annie was ordered to bed on December 4, but was frequently forced to leave it to help in caring for a sick, elderly aunt who lived with the family. Because Annie looked so well and performed her chores with her usual smile, everyone thought she was perhaps not so sick as they had been told. In spite of her pain, Annie cared for this troublesome aunt. After the aunt died, Annie's sister told her, "Dad is glad that now, after the death of Auntie, the family lives in peace." Annie thought for a moment and then replied, "Yes, our good God gave us Auntie to help us practice self-control and strengthen ourselves in virtue, but now that opportunity will be lost to us."

Annie had always felt herself called to the vocation of a cloistered Carmelite, but this life was not possible for her. However, after permission was granted, with a dispensation from the canonical age, her spiritual director admitted her to the Third Order Secular of Carmel. She was soon allowed to make private vows on February 7, 1941.

Months later, on the day of her death, Annie apparently had a glimpse of the other world, since she exclaimed with a smile, "How beautiful it all is . . . I wouldn't trade places with anyone." Then, after kissing her crucifix, she whispered, "My heart is beating for Jesus. I love Him so much . . . I trust . . . Carmel." Annie then died in the peace of God. She was almost 18 years old.

20. Venerable Antonietta (Nennolina) Meo (1930-1937)

ENNOLINA, as she was affectionately called, lived only seven years, but during that time she taught us valuable lessons on how to love God in simple, childlike ways. Nennolina was born into a prosperous and virtuous family of Rome on December 15, 1930. She is described by her family as being "a happy, vivacious, and mischievous child, as are all children her age." When she was in kindergarten, the nuns described her as being in "perpetual motion." But she was a normal child in all respects.

Nennolina was not yet five years old when a swelling was noticed on her left knee. Because of all her activities, it was thought that she had injured it in a fall; but when the swelling grew larger, she was taken to a doctor, who gave an incorrect diagnosis. For reasons only he knew, the child was subjected to injections of iodine. As all children would, Nennolina cried and complained; but when her mother suggested that she think of the sufferings of Jesus, the child bore the pains quietly.

Another doctor correctly diagnosed the problem as cancer of the bone. Because of the delay caused by the first diagnosis, the surgeon could do nothing else to save the life of the child but to amputate her leg. Painful procedures followed, in addition to the fitting of an orthopedic apparatus. Sometime afterward, the doctor described Nennolina's behavior in this way: "She bore the surgical intervention with uncommon fortitude and with joy, always maintaining herself in a joyful attitude, really

47

unusual for a child of her age."

Just a few months later, Nennolina suffered from tonsillitis. While recuperating, she began dictating little messages to Jesus, which she called "poetries." Her mother explained, "I took the first piece of paper that happened to be at hand, and I began to write under dictation, smiling indulgently at what she dictated with so much simplicity and care." Since the mother at first thought them of little importance, some of the earlier poetries were lost; but 177 of them have survived, of which 158 were later published in a book.

When Padre Orlandi visited the child and asked her questions from the catechism, the youngster explained the answers in her own words so clearly and completely that the priest suggested that she receive her First Holy Communion earlier than usual. This began Nennolina's intimate conversations with Jesus, which included words such as: "Dear Jesus, I went for a walk today, and I went to my nuns and I told them that I want to make my First Communion at Christmas. Jesus, You come soon into my heart so I can hold You strongly, and I will kiss You. Jesus, I want You to stay always in my heart."

Another time she dictated: "Dear Jesus, I want You so much. I want to repeat it that I want You so much. I give You my heart. Dear Madonnina, you are so good. You take my heart and hand it to Jesus . . . My good Jesus, give me some souls, give me so many. I ask gladly. I ask You because You make me become good so I can come with you to Heaven."

When she returned to school, Nennolina learned how to use a pen. She signed her dictated letters, "Antonietta and Jesus." Then she wrote, "My dear Jesus, I have learned to do it [use the pen], so soon I will write You by myself"—which she did.

After receiving the Sacrament of Confirmation, Nennolina's condition became progressively worse. She became weak and developed a cough; but in spite of pain, she always wanted to recite her usual morning and evening prayers and her daily devotions. These consisted mainly of the recitation of the holy Rosary and of novenas which she made for the conversion of sinners and for the souls in Purgatory.

One of the poetries which the child dictated to her mother reached Pope Pius XII by way of a professor who had been called in for a consultation regarding Nennolina's medical situation. After reading the following note, the professor felt that the Holy Father should see it; and since he was a friend of the Pope, he brought the note to him.

The note read: "Dear crucified Jesus, I want You so much and I love You so much. I want to be with You on Calvary, and I suffer with joy because I know I am on Calvary. Dear Jesus, I thank You that You have sent me this illness because it is a means to arrive in Heaven . . . Dear Jesus, tell Padre God that I also love Him so much. Dear Jesus, give me the strength to bear these pains that I offer You for sinners . . . Dear Jesus, tell the Holy Spirit that illuminates me of love and gives me the seven gifts. Dear Jesus, tell the Madonnina that I love her so much and I want to be near her on Calvary because I want to be Your victim of love. Dear Jesus, I want to repeat that I love You so much. My good Jesus, I recommend to You my spiritual father and [ask that You] give him necessary graces. . . . Your child sends you so many kisses."

The following day, an envoy from the Pope arrived to present Nennolina with the Apostolic Blessing. The family was told that the Holy Father had been touched by her note and that he recommended himself to the child's prayers.

Nennolina's condition became increasingly worse with the extraction of fluid from her lungs and the adjustment of three ribs under a local anesthetic. The child grimaced from the pain, but never cried or complained. Afterwards, Nennolina announced that she would be in Heaven in ten days.

Large tumors had developed that compressed her lungs, causing suffocation and irritation of the throat. The cancer then progressed to the brain, to a hand and to a foot.

After a time Nennolina became so placid, and she accepted the various procedures so willingly and pleasantly, that her mother asked the doctor if the child's pains had ceased. The doctor replied, "But lady, what do you ask . . . her pains are atrocious."

Exactly ten days later, as Nennolina had predicted, she died on July 3, 1937. She was exactly six years, six months and 19 days old.

After her death the question arose: can a child not yet seven years old reach such a degree of sanctity as to be considered for the honors of the altar? The Congregation for the Causes of Saints studied the matter very carefully and determined that children can attain heroic sanctity and can be considered for canonization.

Soon after Nennolina's death, biographies of her were published which enjoyed wide circulation. Her sanctity was soon recognized by archdiocesan officials, who then permitted the examination of her cause for beatification. Pope Benedict XVI signed a decree on December 17, 2007 recognizing that she had lived the Christian virtues heroically. The Pope declared that Antonietta Meo had "reached the summit of Christian perfection and is an example of holiness for all children."

21. SAINT APOLLONIA (d. 249)

IN a letter written by St. Dionysius of Alexandria, he relates that in the city of Alexandria, a well-known poet who prophesied calamities was successful in introducing a harsh persecution against the Christians. Many of every age were victims of torture, including an elderly man named Metras, who was beaten with reeds and stoned to death. St. Dionysius also tells of a woman called Quinta who refused to worship an idol; she was dragged by her heels over sharp pebbles, cruelly scourged, and then stoned to death. A holy man named Serapion was tortured in his own house with great brutality. After having his bones broken, he was thrown headlong from the top of his house onto the pavement below.

Countless others were treated in various sadistic ways, including St. Apollonia, who was an elderly "deaconess." She received blows to the face so severe that many of her teeth were knocked out. To complete the extractions, the rest of her teeth were removed with pincers. The persecutors then lit a great fire outside the city and threatened to cast her into it unless she uttered certain irreverent words. She begged for a moment's delay to consider the proposal, then, to convince her persecutors that her sacrifice was perfectly voluntary, she leaped into the flames of her own accord.

To explain her actions, St. Augustine reasons that she apparently acted under the inspiration of the Holy Spirit; otherwise, it would have been unlawful for her to have brought about her own death in that way.

St. Apollonia is invoked by those suffering toothache and all dental diseases. She is pictured in art holding a tooth held by a pair of pincers, or holding a golden tooth suspended on a neck chain.

St. Dionysius mentions in his letter to Fabius, Bishop of Antioch, that he had heard of none who had abandoned the Catholic Faith during this persecution.

22. SAINT BENEDICT JOSEPH LABRE (d. 1783)

S T. BENEDICT Joseph Labre was the eldest of 15 children born to a local shopkeeper in Amiettes, a village in the diocese of Boulogne-sur-Mer, France. From his earliest years he was given to prayer, and for this reason he was sent to his uncle, a parish priest of Erin, for his studies. Feeling attracted to the religious life, he sought out the most austere monastery and entered the Trappist Order at the age of 18. But his health proved to be too delicate for their way of life, so he returned home. Next he tried the Carthusians, and then the Cistercians, in both of which attempts he was again disappointed. Having spent a little time in each of these monasteries, he found himself unsuited for community life.

Realizing that the cloister was not meant for him, Benedict decided to follow the example of the many Saints who had embarked on lives of pilgrimage. This led him to travel to shrines in France, Switzerland, Italy, Germany and Spain, often visiting them four or five times. While visiting these shrines, he became an inspiration to many by his pious and reverential demeanor. After he became well known, he once spent so much time in contemplation before a crucifix that a local artist was able to paint the portrait that has preserved the Saint's likeness for us.

Benedict's manner of life would be considered somewhat eccentric by comparison to the lifestyle of most people then or now. Traveling on foot, he slept in the open upon the bare ground and gave away the alms that were given to him. He ate scraps of discarded food, and in time his clothes became thread-bare. His shoes were in a pitiful state, and he carried only a sack and a few books. As a means of mortification, he decided upon an unusual sacrifice. According to Fr. Alban Butler, "Benedict Joseph carried his neglect of his body to a degree that was more galling than any hair shirt, besides earning the contempt which he actually desired." This mortification consisted of voluntarily remaining unwashed, with the result that his body become covered with lice.

About the year 1770, Benedict's pilgrimages ceased, and he remained in Rome. His nights were now spent in the ruins of the Colosseum, and his days in the various churches of the city. He always attended churches that were observing the Forty Hours Devotion, so that the Romans nicknamed him "the Saint of the Forty Hours."

Increasing health problems forced Benedict to enter a hospice for the poor. There he continued his acts of charity by always being the last to be served, by giving his food to those he considered more hungry than himself, and by helping those in need.

During Lent of 1783, after catching a cold that gave him a violent cough, he still maintained his pious practices; but eventually he was forced to accept the hospitality of a butcher, who took Benedict Joseph into his home. There the holy wanderer received the Last Sacraments and died peacefully. As soon as news of his death was made known, children in the streets were heard to cry out, "The Saint is dead!" This was a cry that was repeated throughout the city.

St. Benedict Joseph's holiness became well known throughout Europe, where he was known as the "Beggar of Rome." One of his confessors, during the last years of Benedict Joseph's life, wrote a biography of the Saint that was widely distributed.

23. SERVANT OF GOD BERNARD LEHNER
(1930-1944)

*B*ORN in Herrngiersdorf, Germany, Bernard realized early in life that he was called to a religious vocation, so that by the age of 13 he was attending the seminary school in Regensburg. Unfortunately, his studies were interrupted when he contracted septic diphtheria. In the hospital he seemed to improve, but around Christmas time his condition deteriorated with the onset of paralysis.

All were amazed at young Bernard's willingness to accept bitter medicine and various medical procedures without complaint. He accepted all as a sacrifice for the saving of souls and the good of the Church. In spite of pain, he cheerfully greeted everyone and accepted many requests for prayers. His serene courage in the face of pain and medical complications amazed so many that people considered him a saint.

Bernard suffered intensely for ten weeks. Then, when he realized that he was about to die, he asked for the Last Anointing, telling everyone, "I will soon die, but do not cry, since I am going to Heaven."

On January 24, 1944, fully conscious and surrounded by family and friends, Bernard contentedly entered eternity.

Four years later, in 1948, the case of Bernard Lehner was studied by the local Archbishop, who opened the process for the boy's beatification.

The remains of this young Servant of God are found in the local church, where the citizens extol Bernard's saintly life.

24. SAINT BERNARDINE OF SIENA
(d. 1444)

KNOWN as the Apostle of the Holy Name, St. Bernardine was born in the Tuscan town of Massa Maritima, where his father occupied the post of governor. Orphaned at the age of seven, he was raised by a maternal aunt and received from her his earliest training in virtue. Four years later, he was placed in a school in Siena, where he excelled in his courses. He was noted for his merry disposition, his sweetness, his patience and courtesy.

At the age of 17, Bernardine was enrolled in the Confraternity of Our Lady and pledged himself to certain devotional practices, as well as to the relief of the sick. When Siena was visited by the plague in 1400, he aided the sufferers during the four months that the plague persisted. He escaped the disease and entered the Monastery of San Francesco in Siena and thereafter was sent to the Monastery of Colombaio, where the Rule of St. Francis was more strictly observed.

Ordained a priest, Bernardine soon found difficulty in delivering sermons and in communicating with others because of a hoarseness in his throat. But subsequently, due to fervent prayers offered to Our Lady, his voice became singularly clear and penetrating.

St. Bernardine then began his missionary travels throughout Italy, preaching and exhorting everyone to lives of virtue. He soon attracted multitudes who, out of reverence for him, tried to kiss his hand. To avoid this, the Saint produced a tablet upon which he had written the letters I.H.S., surrounded by rays, which he offered for the people's devotion. In this way he developed reverence for the Holy Name of Jesus.

In the city of his birth, during the Lenten season of 1444, Bernardine preached for 50 consecutive days and then bid farewell. He died when almost 64 years of age, 42 of which had been spent as a religious. He was canonized within six years of his death, due to the many miracles performed at his tomb in Aquila.

25. Saint Camillus de Lellis
(1550-1614)

AS a child, Camillus proved to be somewhat of a disappointment to his parents since he was exceedingly vivacious and troublesome, an instigator and a participant in many street brawls, a frequent truant from school, and a compulsive gambler. By the age of 13, he was so tall that he towered over those of his age and might have been considered a giant.

Since his father was a captain and commander of the local garrison, Camillus, at the age of 19, joined him in the army to fight against the Turks at Lepanto. He also saw action in Dalmatia and Africa. During this time he developed an ulcerated leg, for which he sought treatment in the Hospital of St. James in Rome.

At the time of his discharge Camillus had gambled away his inheritance and his weapons, and, since he had little inclination for work, he became a beggar. But he was eventually offered a job as a stonemason, which brought him into contact with the Capuchin Fathers, who counseled him into a complete reform.

Camillus twice entered the monastery, but each time the recurring ulceration of his leg caused his dismissal. He again applied for treatment at the Hospital of St. James in Rome, but his condition proved to be a lifelong affliction that was resistant to treatment.

Camillus remained at the hospital, caring for patients, until he became dissatisfied with the servants' lack of co-operation and constant unfaithfulness to duty. It was then that he began establishing an Order whose members were to bind themselves, by a fourth vow, to the charitable care of the sick and dying.

With the encouragement of his confessor, St. Philip Neri, Camillus began studying for the priesthood. He was ordained on June 10, 1584.

In addition to his diseased leg, the Saint, during the last years of his life, endured a painful rupture, frequent renal colic, and spasmodic stomach pains—yet he managed to visit all the institutions for the sick and dying that he had established throughout Italy. Then he returned to Rome to prepare for his death, which took place on July 14, 1614.

The symbol of the Red Cross, which represents mercy and help to persons in need, is usually thought to have originated in recent times, but it was actually first used by St. Camillus when he founded the Order of Ministers of the Sick. He received Papal approval for his Order, with the added permission for the members to wear a large red cross on the front of their black habits. The Order the Saint founded is now known as the Order of St. Camillus, or simply the Camillians. The Order is found in the United States, Canada, Europe, South America and many other countries.

Camillus de Lellis was canonized in 1746 by Pope Benedict XIV. Along with St. John of God, his Spanish counterpart, St. Camillus has been given a triple designation by Pope Leo XIII and Pope Pius XI as the patron of the sick, of nurses, and of hospitals.

26. Blessed Carlos Manuel Rodriguez
(1918-1963)

CARLOS was born into a deeply religious family in Caguas, Puerto Rico in 1918. Life with his brother and three sisters was serene and normal. Two of his sisters married, and the third became a Carmelite nun. His only brother became a Benedictine priest and was the first Puerto Rican to become the abbot of a monastery.

Carlos began school at the age of six and completed his primary studies with success, having received first prize for scholastic achievement and also a special prize for religion. While attending his first year of high school, Carlos experienced the first symptoms of a condition that would gradually increase in severity until it would eventually claim his life: ulcerative colitis. He completed high school, with various interruptions, in 1939, after completing both commercial and general programs. To support himself, Carlos worked at clerical jobs, but his main interest was the apostolate of making Christ known and loved as he knew and loved Him.

Carlos attempted formal studies at the University of Puerto Rico, but he missed many days for health reasons. Even so, his grades were extraordinary, since he was coached by a friend on the subjects that he missed during his long absences. Carlos never finished college but he continued his education on his own, reading voraciously.

Although very virtuous, Carlos never expressed a desire to become a priest. Instead, he worked as an office clerk at the

60

Agriculture Experiment Station in Caguas, which was part of the University of Puerto Rico. He spent his free time dispensing Catholic materials, editing Catholic journals, arranging student instructional meetings, writing Catholic articles and giving lectures about the Faith.

Despite his illness, he organized and directed a group of men at the university, to whom he gave lectures. One of his "disciples" was a renowned professor who said, "This young man is what my good friend Gabriela Mistral used to call a 'child of the Holy Spirit.'" Carlos was also the leader of another group of men in Caguas. During their meetings he answered questions concerning faith and morals. He translated into English various Spanish books of devotion, and he organized other groups of men, as well as the *Te Deum Laudamus* choir. Carlos taught many how to use the missal when Mass was still being universally offered in Latin. He also began a publication, *Liturgy and Christian Culture,* for which he paid most of the expenses. He accomplished all this while maintaining a steady clerical job and feeling ill most of the time.

Other organizations were established and various successful endeavors were credited to Carlos, but all this came to a close during the early part of 1963 when his face showed unmistakable signs of ill health and he became extremely tired. He underwent tests, which revealed severe anemia and a rectal mass. Painful biopsies were taken of the mass, which was said to be non-malignant. For four months nothing was done, but then the test proved to have been incorrect: the mass was in fact cancerous.

Finally, Carlos underwent surgery. Without notifying him of their plans, the doctors prepared him for a radical, seven-hour operation. The doctors confirmed Carlos' cancer, and it was necessary for them to remove numerous lymph nodes and perform a colostomy. The results of his surgery were a great shock to Carlos, especially the colostomy, which not only caused painful skin irritation but also a loss of dignity and privacy. Carlos was now suffering from end-stage rectal cancer.

Carlos was moved to a private dispensary, where he confided to his doctor: "I suffer not so much for myself as for so many other sick people who have no one to take care of them when they ask for something so basic as a glass of water." Carlos never complained; instead, he begged pardon for causing so much inconvenience. Doctors later found tumors in his liver and throughout the rest of his body. There was no hope for recovery. Without being told, Carlos understood and remained silent in recollection.

Added to the physical pain was his spiritual distress, which his confessor considered to be the "Dark Night of the Soul" as described by St. John of the Cross. Carlos received Holy Communion every day, and eventually the Dark Night was lifted. He predicted that he would die on July 13. He lapsed into a coma and died on the day predicted. He was 44 years old.

Carlos' process for beatification was one of the shortest in recent history. It was initiated in 1992, he was declared Venerable in 1997 and beatified on April 29, 2001.

27. SAINT CHARLES LWANGA AND COMPANIONS (d. 1885-1887)

WHEN Mwanga became King of the country of Uganda in Africa, he was only 18 years old. The former king, his father, had previously expelled the White Fathers from the territory, but Mwanga had always liked "the praying ones," and he invited them to return.

For a time, peace was restored, and many accepted the Catholic Faith. The converts included Charles Lwanga, who was recognized as the strongest athlete of the court. He was also regarded as "the most handsome man of the kingdom of Uganda." Charles, who had been a page in the previous court, now became the chief of the royal pages.

Unfortunately, King Mwanga had as his chief assistant Katikiro, who had been the chief assistant to the previous king. He disliked the priests and their Christian (Catholic) followers; gradually, by devising false rumors, he convinced the young king that the Christians were plotting against him. King Mwanga began to regret recalling the missionaries, and he became a staunch enemy of the Christians. One day he ordered that all the Christian boy pages should be found out and killed as punishment.

That night, while the drums sounded as a signal for the assembly of the executions, Charles Lwanga gathered together all the pages and other Christians. When asked the next morning if they wanted to renounce the Catholic Faith, all refused. All the Christians were then condemned to death by fire and were forced to walk 17 miles to the place of execution. Along the way, other Christians joined them voluntarily.

According to a traditional procedure, the chief executioners had the right to reserve for themselves one of the condemned whom they could torture as they pleased. Chosen for this special treatment was Charles Lwanga, who told his companions as he left them, "I shall see you very soon. Very shortly I shall join you in Heaven."

When one of the little martyrs saw that fires were being readied, he said to one of the guards, "You can very well burn my body, but you cannot burn my soul, for it belongs to God." Charles Lwanga stood aside while his companions were placed on reed mats that were then rolled around their bodies. Each was then enclosed in a bundle of wood which was securely tied about him. All were burned alive.

When Charles saw that a special pyre was being prepared for him, he asked to be untied so that he could help in arranging the place of torture. In a cheerful and peaceful manner, Charles arranged the wood and sticks and then lay down upon them. It was then announced that, unlike the others, who had been killed quickly, Charles would be burned over a slow fire. Charles answered bravely that he was very glad to die for the True Faith.

With flames licking at his feet, Charles stiffened, but did not utter a single cry. The torture lasted a long time, with Charles twisting under the pain, but he remained ever faithful to his religion. Charles was heard to moan repeatedly, *Katonda!*—"O my God!"

During the march to the place of execution, three prisoners were set free, for reasons unknown. One of these, Denis Kamyuka, heard one of the executioners say on his return to the village, "We have killed many men in our time, but never such as these! The others did nothing but moan and weep, but these prayed right to the end."

A few days later, some Christians from a nearby village went secretly to the place of execution and collected a few charred bones and ashes. These were later deposited in a reliquary which is now kept in the Cathedral of St. Mary of Rubaga. This church is located on the very place where the palace of the king once stood.

The details of the heroic death of Charles Lwanga and his 21 companions became well-known, due to the testimony of Denis Kamyuka, who had been released during the death march. During the ecclesiastical inquiry, Denis repeated the names of the martyrs and related the details that had surrounded their deaths. The Martyrs of Uganda were eventually canonized by Pope Paul VI on June 22, 1964.

St. Charles Lwanga has been designated the Patron of the African Youth of Catholic Action. He might well serve also as a patron of those who have suffered from fire.

28. BLESSED CHIARA LUCE BADANO
(1971-1990)

ER pious parents, Ruggero and Maria Teresa Badano, were married 11 years before Chiara arrived on October 29, 1971 in Sassello, Italy. She was their only child. She was a beautiful and pleasant little girl and loved attending religion classes. By the age of nine she was eager to start exercising her spirit of charity by joining a church group whose meetings and activities were designed for children her age. She was especially attracted to helping the elderly, and she assisted them and her classmates as much as she could.

Chiara Luce was very athletic and particularly loved to play tennis. It was during one of her practice sessions that she felt a severe pain in her shoulder. When the pain continued and grew worse, she was diagnosed as having osteosarcoma with metastasis, a very painful and deadly form of cancer. She and her parents accepted the news courageously, with Chiara declaring that the illness was the will of God.

Chiara underwent two operations, followed by chemotherapy. She began losing her hair but was not the least upset or concerned. As each clump fell, she said, "For You, Jesus." When she lost the use of her legs, she remarked, "If I had to choose between walking again or going to Heaven, I would choose Heaven without hesitation."

Chiara always refused morphine to reduce the pain, saying that she wanted to remain clear-headed so that she could offer her pains to Jesus. She was heard to remark, "I want to share a little bit of His cross with Him." Another time she said, "What is this pain in comparison with the nails in the hands of Jesus?"

After recovering from a severe hemorrhage in July of 1989, Chiara Luce realized the end was near, and she cautioned her parents not to cry. "At the funeral," she said, "I don't want people to cry, I want them to sing." She referred to her funeral as the wedding feast and asked to be dressed as a bride. She chose the songs and even the readings for her funeral Mass. She recommended to her mother, "When you are dressing me, think: Chiara Luce now sees Jesus."

All were impressed with Chiara's willing acceptance of death and her deep spirituality. When asked why her eyes seemed so intensely luminous, she replied, "I try to love Jesus a lot!"

During the last moments of her life she whispered, "Goodbye, Mom. Be happy because I'm very happy." She died on October 7, 1990 at the age of 18. The funeral was conducted by the local bishop in the presence of more than 2,000 people. Chiara was beatified on September 25, 2010.

29. Venerable Cleonilde Guerra
(1922-1949)

*B*ORN in San Potito (Ravenna), Italy, Cleonilde was somewhat sickly from early childhood after being stricken with pneumonia, but even as a child she bore her pain in silence.

She loved to read, and she became familiar with the Gospels and the lives of the Saints, especially the lives of St. Thérèse of Lisieux and St. Gemma Galgani. Encouraged by her parish priest, she was attracted to Christian virtues and was active in parish activities.

Cleonilde felt drawn to the religious life when she was 16, but she did not enter because of the objection of her father. However, she did maintain a close relationship with the Handmaids of the Sacred Heart of the Dying Jesus. She was encouraged by these nuns in her vocation, and she eventually entered the Order when she was 21. A recurrence of her childhood ailment, however, made it necessary for her to leave—which she did with great disappointment.

Cleonilde's failure to continue the religious life brought on a deep depression, which she suffered until a priest named Father Savorini convinced her that the religious life was not God's Will for her. After her mind was restored to peace, Cleonilde began once again to work for the parish and became a militant worker in Catholic Action.

The return of the people to San Potito after World War II encouraged Cleonilde to work untiringly in her parish for the moral and spiritual regeneration of the people. She loved to teach and did so by preparing children for their First Holy Communion and their reception of the Sacrament of Confirmation.

Cleonilde died at San Potito on May 19, 1949, with a reputation of great holiness. She was 27. The petition for her beatification has been accepted by the Congregation for the Causes of Saints. Her heroic virtue was declared in 2007.

30. Venerable Concepta Bertoli
(1908-1956)

CONCEPTA was a healthy little girl when she was born on April 14, 1908 in the village of Mereto di Tomba, near the city of Udine in northeastern Italy. Her first 16 years were spent happily in school and in helping in the fields, but toward the end of her 16th year, she developed a type of arthritis that began to deform her body. Gradually she became completely immobilized. Her teeth became clenched and her jaws locked, so that the only nourishment she could take was in liquid form. Severe arthritis developed in her body and twisted it into an awkward position, so that for the next 31 years, Concepta remained in that position, experiencing pain and extreme discomfort. She endured her condition so well, without complaint, that she was referred to by the villagers as a living crucifix.

Concepta accepted her condition as the Will of God and became a Franciscan tertiary in 1940. Her physical condition became even more severe ten years later when she became completely blind, a condition that lasted for the rest of her life.

Concepta was so convinced that her condition was the Will of God and that she was experiencing pain as did Jesus on Calvary, that she revealed: "I don't have enough breath to thank the Lord, who has put me under these conditions. I can do so much good here on my bed. The Lord entrusts to each a place and a mission. To me He has given this bed. I am happy. Suffering without resignation is awful; but, if there is resignation, pain is nothing." In her youth she had wanted to be a missionary, but now she claimed, "I am a missionary of pain."

When Concepta was 30 years old she was taken on a stretcher to Lourdes, where she asked for the grace to endure her sufferings and for the grace to communicate a little better, since the position of her teeth and the rigidity of her jaws prevented clear speech.

Two years later she was taken to the Holy House of Loreto. There was some speculation at the time that her blindness had been temporarily lifted during this visit, but afterward she commented, "I have lost the sight of the eyes, but I have the eyes of faith."

When the 25th anniversary of the onset of her sufferings was approaching, Concepta wanted it to be observed in a special way. It was, with the ringing of church bells and a beautiful Holy Mass.

Concepta said that she felt she would die during the year 1956. She added, "But I am happy because I will go with the Lord." She died on March 11 of that year and was buried in the parish church. Her tomb has an inscription stating that her pains were offered to God for priests, missionaries and sinners. It also mentions that Concepta was always pleasant and was blessed by God.

The informative process for the cause of her beatification was begun in 1969, only 13 years after her death. The cause advanced in 1994, and on April 24, 2001, Concepta Bertoli was declared Venerable by the Congregation for the Causes of Saints.

31. Saint Damien Joseph de Veuster
(1840-1889)

AMIEN was born Joseph de Veuster in Tremeloo, Belgium, and received the name Damien after his entrance into the novitiate of the Fathers of the Sacred Hearts of Jesus and Mary of Louvain. After his Ordination, he served as pastor in a comfortable parish in Honolulu on Oahu, Hawaii's main island. When he learned that the approximately 800 lepers on the island of Molokai were without the services of a priest, he promptly volunteered to go to Molokai. Before leaving, he was advised on how to avoid the disease by proper sanitary means. But Damien soon began to minister to the lepers in their hovels, helping them with bandages; and while performing other services, he often came into physical contact with the lepers' skin and body fluids, the very situation against which he had been warned. Personal contact with lepers was unavoidable since he served them as physician, house-builder, sheriff, counselor, undertaker and gravedigger, besides helping them in all manner of charitable endeavors.

Damien had arrived at Molokai in 1873, and within one year he saw in himself the first symptoms of the disease when dry spots began appearing on his feet and legs. Damien had contracted Hansen's disease, or leprosy, as it is better known. After six years the symptoms disappeared, but then they returned with renewed vigor. His sciatic nerve caused excruciating pain which ran from the lower spine down the legs and caused numbness to his feet. The numbness of his feet was so complete that once, after bathing them, he realized that the water was boiling hot only when sores began to appear. When leprous marks started appearing on his face, he wrote in a letter, "Soon I will be disfigured entirely. Having no doubts about the true nature of my disease, I am calm, resigned and very happy in the midst of my people. God certainly knows what is best for my sanctification and I gladly repeat: 'Thy will be done!'"

Later Fr. Damien wrote, "I'm having a hard time saying Mass; I have to sit down to preach; and since I can no longer walk, I ride around in a wagon. So, in the midst of our patients, I myself am playing the part of a sick man."

When asked by his superiors if he wanted to leave for medical treatment, the priest declined, saying that he refused to leave his flock and abandon his work. Damien had become a veritable martyr for the sake of charity and the welfare of the abandoned sick.

Damien's face was badly covered with leprosy when he died on April 15, 1889. Although he had expressed the desire to remain buried among the lepers' graves on Molokai, his body was returned to his native land in 1936. He was declared Venerable in 1977, beatified on June 4, 1995 and canonized by Pope Benedict XVI on October 11, 2009.

32. SAINT DROGO (d. 1186)

ROGO became an orphan only moments after his birth. His father had died shortly before he was born, and his mother died during childbirth. When he was old enough to realize that his mother's life had been sacrificed for his own, he went into a deep depression, accusing himself bitterly. Thankfully, he learned to trust in the wisdom of God and accepted his mother's death as the will of the Almighty.

Drogo was 18 when he decided to follow Our Lord's example of complete poverty. He began his penitential life by abandoning his home, his country and his inheritance. He journeyed through several countries, visiting holy places and receiving many spiritual blessings, which aided him in advancing in the interior life. After a time he decided to settle down; he did so at Sebourg, near Valenciennes, France.

There he was hired as a shepherd, and he became so well known for his virtues that many regarded him as a saint. It was noticed by the villagers that while Drogo was tending his flocks in the fields, he was also seen attending Mass in the village church. This gift of bilocation gave rise to a local saying: "Not being St. Drogo, I cannot be in two places at the same time."

After six years of tending sheep, Drogo resumed his pilgrimages. It is said that he visited Rome on nine occasions, but the last visit ended in a pathetic manner.

The physical condition that made it impossible for Drogo to continue traveling has been described as a "peculiarly repulsive hernia that could not be hidden." In an effort to shield himself from his neighbors, in order not to offend them by his appearance, Drogo retired to a cell that had been built against the church. Through a small window he was able to assist at Mass without entering the body of the church. He was fed and cared for through the generosity of those who admired his virtues and pitied his condition. He spent 40 years in his small room beside the church, praying, fasting, and suffering greatly from his affliction.

When Drogo died at the age of 84, his tomb became a favorite place of pilgrimage. He is regarded as the patron of shepherds and is invoked by those who suffer from hernia.

33. SERVANT OF GOD
ELISABETTA TASCA SERENA (1899-1978)

IN ADDITION to St. Gianna Beretta Molla, whose life story is included in this book, another opponent of abortion is this Servant of God, Elisabetta Tasca Serena, who was blessed with 12 children.

Elisabetta herself was born the last of seven children in an old country house in San Zenone of Ezzelini near Treviso in northern Italy. Her life was difficult and poor from the start. At the time of her birth, and in the area where she was born, there were two main social groups, the squires and the middle class. The squires owned large tracts of land and great herds of livestock; the middle class worked the land for them. Elisabetta's family was very poor, and the conditions under which they lived were often austere.

As a child, Elisabetta was vivacious, very active, and very talented in that she crocheted beautiful articles that she sold or gave as gifts. She often did this work while tending animals in the fields. Often she brought groups of small boys with her to pasture, where she repeated to them the sermons she had heard. One of the boys reported when he was grown: "I went gladly to the pasture with Elisabetta, because she told me the sacred history and the lives of the Saints. One day she told us the life story of St. Maria Goretti and how strongly we must respect the virtue of purity. During my long life, I have always remembered the words of Elisabetta, so much they have been engraved in my heart."

Elisabetta was 20 when she began to consider an offer of marriage made by a young man, Joseph Serena. Uncertain if he was the young man God had chosen for her, she prayed the Rosary. At the Third Joyful Mystery, she received an answer to her prayer. The two were married on April 6, 1921. Elisabetta moved into the house of her in-laws, and it was there that her children were born. She proved to be a joy to the numerous members of the family. "She brought song, sincere and intelligent affection to her husband, and a great Christian culture."

When the children began arriving one after the other, the doctor discovered a serious physical problem and twice suggested that Elisabetta might want to abort the babies rather than face the serious risk of death. Elisabetta quickly responded: "Never abortion in my house. If I have to die, it is the Will of God . . . My children are my most beautiful flowers, and I thank the Lord that He wanted them to grow in my garden."

Some of Elisabetta's pregnancies were very difficult, with long convalescent periods. Many years later, when looking upon her 12 children, she was known to have said, "I live in serenity. Those mothers that have killed their children through abortion—how do they live?" Of her 12 children, eight were happily married, two became priests and two became nuns.

Elisabetta attended Mass every day, received the Sacraments, was involved in parish activities, taught catechism and sang in the choir—in addition to all the chores required of her in caring for her large family.

When her husband became ill, she took care of him for eight years, until his death. Afterward, without his income, people were curious as to how she clothed so many children in the midst of poverty. She replied that many people gave her clothes that their own children had outgrown. She served for a time as a nanny and thus made a little money; when the children were older, the family bought clothes with money they had made from gleaning wheat from reaped fields. They also sold rabbits and made food products which they sold.

During her later years, Elisabetta continued to attend daily Mass. Once she told a neighbor, "After receiving Holy Communion, I have everything. Yes, with Jesus in my heart I have everything and can go to face my job and the troubles of the day with trust and joy. Be always happy. If inside there is something that makes you suffer, don't lose your courage, and remember Him. It will then pass after a prayer, and then sing! If you knew how many sorrows have passed me by with a song. And so it will be for you. And give to everyone one of your smiles."

Elisabetta's final illness, a lung condition, brought about her death on October 2, 1978. In the hospital she had been stricken with strong pains in the liver and the intestines, which required two urgent operations. She never complained during this illness or during her many difficult pregnancies.

After receiving the Sacraments from one of her priest sons, Elisabetta died peacefully at the age of 79. The funeral took place with 27 priests in attendance. Afterward, when the diocesan process for her beatification was initiated, more than 144 testimonials were received. Written by priests, nuns and lay people, the testimonials told of help extended, good advice given, good example imitated, conversions effected and lessons taught. In view of Elisabetta's virtuous life, the Vatican issued the decree *Positio Super Virtutibus* in 1994, declaring her to be a Servant of God.

34. BLESSED ELIZABETH OF THE TRINITY
(1880-1906)

BETTER known as Elizabeth of the Trinity, Elizabeth Catez was born to Captain Joseph Catez and Marie Catez at a military camp in the diocese of Bourges, France. After her father's death when she was seven, Elizabeth and her sister Marguerite were raised by their mother, who noted that Elizabeth, because she was stubborn and given to fits of rage, would "become either a terror or a saint." This child was quite a problem until the time of her First Holy Communion, when she abruptly decided to change her disposition.

At the age of 14, having heard the word "Carmel" after the reception of Holy Communion, Elizabeth felt called to become a Carmelite nun, having already been acquainted with the Order since childhood. But she was not allowed to enter until her 22nd birthday, in accord with the wishes of her mother. During the intervening years, she dedicated herself to prayer and penance and developed a cheerful disposition. She attended family gatherings and was quite adept at playing the piano, and she often played to entertain her family and friends.

Before her entrance into Carmel, Elizabeth had a long conversation with Father Valee, a Dominican, who explained that the Blessed Trinity dwelt in her soul. Thereafter, she decided to please God by meditating often on the indwelling of the Holy Trinity, often writing about this practice and explaining that "It is wonderful to recall that, except for the vision of seeing God, we possess God as all the Saints in Heaven do . . . He dwells in our souls!" After entering Carmel in 1901 and being professed in 1903, Elizabeth suffered from spiritual dryness and the "dark night of the soul" as explained by St. John of the Cross.

Sometime after her profession, Elizabeth offered herself as a "victim soul" and soon developed Addison's Disease, a hormonal disorder that is accompanied by chronic fatigue, lightheadedness, low blood pressure, nausea, vomiting, diarrhea, weak muscles and spasms. She endured these symptoms until November 9, 1906, when she uttered her dying words, "I am going to Light, to Love, to Life!" She was a mere 26 years old.

The writings of Bl. Elizabeth regarding the indwelling of the Holy Trinity have been studied and commended by a number of outstanding theologians, including Father Philipon, O.P. Elizabeth of the Trinity was beatified by Pope John Paul II on November 25, 1984.

35. SERVANT OF GOD
FAUSTINO PEREZ-MANGLANO (1946-1963)

FAUSTINO was a modern boy, living during the time of Vatican Council II. He was very much an athlete, since he participated in hiking, swimming, camping, sleeping in tents, climbing mountains—and he was especially fond of soccer. For a time he studied judo, and he indulged in a little slang. Faustino would today be considered "well adjusted," and his friends claim that "he was always smiling." He was born in Valencia, Spain, the son of a doctor. One of four children, he was baptized at the same font where St. Vincent Ferrer had also received the Sacrament.

Faustino was always a good boy, but his virtues increased dramatically when he was 13, after he made his first retreat. He was to claim that the retreat "changed my life completely." He began the daily recitation of the Rosary and kept a spiritual diary that reveals his steady progress in virtue. At the same time, being a very active boy in all respects, he loved to keep track of the local Valencia soccer team, and he wrote about the team many times in his diary. One notation reads, "I prayed the Rosary. I went to Communion during recreation . . . I talked ten minutes with Christ about the Zaragoza-Valencia tie [a soccer game] and the missions." Another time he wrote, "I prayed the Rosary and went to Communion. We won the soccer game 10-3. I spoke 10 minutes with Christ . . . "

At the end of November, 1960, Faustino felt a lump under his arm. An operation was performed to remove it. The operation

81

made him very ill and gave him great pain for almost a year. Unable to attend school, he studied at home in between radiation treatments. The diagnosis in early 1961 was frightening: an apparent malignant infection of the lymph glands. After a visit to another doctor and after Faustino experienced sharp pains in the lumbar region, x-rays revealed a vertebra being pressured by a tumor. It was soon revealed that Faustino had a fatal form of Hodgkins' disease.

Because of the treatments, he became bloated and then lost all his hair—a thing of little consequence to him. He was quiet, serious and suffered greatly, but he was never heard to complain.

In his diary, Faustino began to write of his desire to become a Marianist priest. In all, he wrote about his vocation to the religious life 42 times.

Since he was particularly devoted to Our Lady of the Pillar, a devotion beloved of the Marianist Order, Faustino was taken to that shrine in Zaragoza. He was also taken to Lourdes, where he served as a "brancardier" or stretcher-bearer. He did not receive a cure, but he did receive a reserve of energy that helped him.

For a brief time he was able to resume camping, but when the first session of Vatican II began, his illness returned. Phlebitis now affected both his legs, yet he continued to smile. He insisted on attending school, where his classmates saw him smiling even though he had to drag himself from one place to another, bent over like an old man. One friend commented, "What impressed me most was his capacity for suffering. When I found out that they even had to dress him, and that he studied in bed, I was astonished. That was when I realized how much he suffered. He never said, 'I'm in pain today,' and I never noticed it."

Faustino wrote in his diary at this time, "A death with the

Virgin is marvelous. Christ, grant that every day I may be more devoted to Mary. I want to be always intimately united to her. She will help me to die, and I will have the death of a true saint."

Before his death, Faustino's desire to become a Marianist was realized. Permission was received for him to profess vows *in articulo mortis*—basically, in a dying state. He was delighted that his dream had been realized. He was a Marianist after all.

Faustino received Holy Communion every day. He also suffered grievously, with his body greatly swollen. He died in the arms of his mother, while holding a medal of the Blessed Virgin Mary. He was 16 years old. One of the last notations in Faustino's diary reads, "Sanctity is very difficult. But I will try, and who knows if I might achieve it?" Faustino is well on the way to receiving recognition for his sanctity since a cause for his beatification was initiated in 1986.

36. SAINT FRANCIS DE SALES
(1567-1622)

ORN in a castle near Annecy, located in southeastern France, our saint was the first child of noble parents who had been married seven years before his birth. After his arrival the couple welcomed two other sons and one daughter. His brother, John Francis, would later succeed him as Bishop of Geneva. The family eventually consisted of ten other children.

Because his father wanted him to be a lawyer and attain political prominence, Francis was sent to the University of Paris, where he studied for seven years. The saint once remarked, "In Paris I studied many things to please my father and theology to please myself."

Francis also studied at the University of Padua for three years and earned a brilliant degree as a doctor of law. Sometime later, after finding a spiritual director, Francis revealed that since the age of twelve he had carried the hope of one day becoming a priest. Eventually he was ordained. The ordination took place a week before Christmas, on December 18, 1593.

Against the wishes of his father, Francis volunteered to work in the Chablais region, where, by treaty, the territory was legally Catholic but the local authorities were Calvinists who strongly resisted the Catholic Church. More than one attempt was made on the life of the courageous priest. Because conditions made it difficult to teach and counsel in person as he wanted to, the saint began by writing what he called "Meditations" and slipping these tracts under the doors of known Catholics, as well as posting them in public places. Thirty-six years after his death these tracts were collected and published under the title of *Controversies,* and later as *The Catholic Controversy.* This is a work which has been reprinted many times, more recently by TAN Books and Publishers.

Francis labored in the Chablais between the ages of 27 and 31. He was so successful that he was able to report the following to Pope Clement VIII in 1603: "Twelve years ago, heresy was in occupation in 64 parishes. It had invaded everything. Catholicism held not even an inch of territory. Today the Catholic Church in those places spreads its branches everywhere, and with such vigor that heresy can find no room. Before, it was hard to find 100 Catholics within all those parishes taken together; today, it would be just as hard to find 100 heretics . . ."

No doubt because of his success and his many talents and deep spirituality, in 1602 Francis became the Bishop of Geneva, a city which was also dominated by the Calvinist heresy. He was consecrated after refusing several times, and he even declined the office of cardinal.

One of the greatest accomplishments of the saint was the founding of the Order of the Visitation with St. Jane Frances de Chantal. At the time, St. Jane was a widow with four children, the youngest being only six. We are told that after providing for the care of the children, she approached the doorway to leave— and found it necessary to step over the body of her 15-year-old son, who was making a dramatic attempt to dissuade her from leaving for the convent.

St. Francis is the author of two classics of the spiritual life, *An Introduction to the Devout Life* and *Treatise on the Love of God,* both of which have remained popular through the years. Since their publication they have consistently remained bestsellers in many languages. In these works the saint reveals his great love of the Sacred Heart and also of the Blessed Virgin, to whom he had recited a Rosary daily since his youth.

As to the physical troubles of the saint, these are described for us by St. Jane de Chantal herself in a deposition for his beatification. She wrote: "All through the 19 years during which I had the great honor of his acquaintance, I know, both from hearsay and from my own personal observation, that he suffered from all sorts of maladies: from attacks of fever, sore throats and colds, and from internal abdominal weakness which greatly exhausted him and which accompanied him for many years with severe hemorrhage. These ailments increased with his advancing years, and in addition to excruciating pains in the head and body, he suffered from weakness and even open wounds in the legs. He had varicose veins which made walking so difficult and so fatiguing that it was grievous to see him wearily struggling along."

St. Jane added: "Yet in spite of all these sufferings, and many more of which nothing was known, he made no change whatever in his manner of life and so controlled his countenance that he was only known to be ill by his change of color, especially as he never took to his bed except when overtaken by very serious illness."

On December 27, 1622, the saint collapsed after presiding over the exhausting ceremonies for Christmas. His condition was quickly diagnosed by the medical professionals as a brain hemorrhage. Since it was believed at the time that a patient in his condition should not fall asleep, they pinched, rubbed and slapped him in an effort to keep him awake. After this, they applied a plaster of blister beetles and then pressed a red-hot iron against the back of his neck. After other treatments he was returned to his bed, where he died the following day. Of course, the treatments only advanced the sad condition of the exhausted bishop and hastened his death soon afterward.

St. Francis was beatified in 1662 and canonized three years later. He was declared a Doctor of the Church by Pope Pius IX in 1877. Because of his writings, which are still popular today, he was designated by Pope Pius XI as Patron of the Catholic Press.

37. Saint Germaine Cousin
(1579-1601)

URING the process for her beatification, Germaine was described as "a simple maiden, humble and of lowly birth, but so greatly enlightened by the gifts of divine wisdom and understanding, and so remarkable for her transcendent virtues, that she shone like a star, not only in her native France, but also throughout the Catholic Church."

Germaine's father was a poor agricultural laborer of Pibrac, a village ten miles from Toulouse in Southwestern France. Unfortunately, her mother died only months after Germaine's birth. Germaine had difficulties from the moment of her birth. She was born with a right hand that was crippled and powerless. Then, when she was a little older, she developed a scrofulous condition of the neck glands that produced huge swellings which deformed her appearance. One can only wonder what treatment she received from children her age and from adults who avoided her for fear the condition was contagious.

Added to the harsh treatment she received outside the house, Germaine's father, who had no affection for her, took a second wife, who actively disliked the young girl. Germaine was treated harshly by the stepmother, who eventually gave birth to her own children. To be rid of Germaine, she offered the pretext that her young children should be spared contact with Germaine, lest they become infected. The father, having little concern for Germaine, banished her from the house, making it necessary for her to seek shelter in the stable or under the stairs outside the house.

In all kinds of weather the child was made to endure the rigors of a crude, unheated stable or the inadequate shelter of the stairs. Her food, which was grudgingly given her, consisted of scraps of bread and the leftovers from the plates of the other children. When the parents decided she was old enough, she was sent to tend the sheep in the pastures. She was destined to remain a shepherdess for the rest of her life.

Despite the ill-treatment she received, Germaine accepted everything with perfect resignation and simplicity of heart. This was used by God to advance her in the spiritual life. While tending the flocks in the quiet fields, she communed with her divine Creator. She was devoted to the Rosary, which she recited with great care, and she attended Mass every day and received the Eucharist as often as permitted.

Germaine never engaged in the social life of the peasants or mixed with girls of her own age—who were apparently repulsed by her deformity. However, she did take pleasure in instructing children in the truths of the Catholic Faith and in encouraging them in the love of God.

On seeing the treatment given to Germaine by her parents, the neighbors likewise dealt her a generous helping of intolerance. However, they began to change their attitude when strange reports started circulating about her. It was revealed that when Germaine left her flock of sheep to attend Mass, the sheep never left the crook she had thrust into the ground and that, although unattended, they were never harassed by the wolves that lurked in the nearby forest. It was also reported that a swollen stream parted, much like the Red Sea in the time of Moses, allowing Germaine to cross the stream on her way to Mass.

The villagers soon began to treat Germaine with courtesy, claiming that the young girl was a saint. The father and step-

mother also relented and offered to take her into the house, but
Germaine declined their offer, preferring to live as before.

Germaine was found one morning lying dead on her straw
mat under the stairs. She was only 22 years old. Because of her
saintly conduct and the miracles witnessed by the villagers, the
body of the little shepherdess was buried in the church of Pibrac
where she had so often attended the Holy Sacrifice of the Mass.
Forty-three years after her death, two church workers opened
the vault to make room for another burial and found the body
of a beautiful young girl lying in a state of perfect preservation.
The older villagers recognized Germaine's body immediately by
the crippled arm and the scrofulous wounds on the neck. A tool
used by one of the men slipped, injuring the nose of the body,
which immediately began to bleed.

This wonder, together with many miracles of healing,
prompted the initiation of a cause for her beatification. In 1850
more than 400 miracles of extraordinary graces and healings
were classified. Germaine was eventually canonized on June 29,
1867 by Pope Pius IX. The body that had remained incorrupt
for many years was deliberately destroyed in 1795 during the
French Revolution, so that now only a few relics remain.

38. SAINT GIANNA BERETTA MOLLA
(1922-1962)

THE family into which Gianna Beretta was born in 1922 was an extraordinary one. Both parents were Third Order Franciscans who taught their children to live simply, frugally, and with fraternal joy. One of the children, who later became a priest, said that they "lived an intense life of piety and evangelical mortification, renouncing even exteriorly all that was superfluous." Both parents attended daily Mass with their children, and in the evening the Rosary was recited, followed by happy and animated conversation. A daughter added, "Never did a strong or uncontrolled word disturb the serenity of the family, never was there a reproof from the mother without the support of the father . . . the atmosphere of the home was permeated with serenity and peace." This was all the more remarkable since there were 13 children in the family.

One of her early teachers recalled that Gianna had a sweet character: "She was always smiling. I never heard a word of annoyance, fatigue or rebellion cross her lips. . . . The fulfillment of her duties at home, in school, in society were for her a sacred duty. Diligent and committed to her studies, she was a model of respect and discipline."

Gianna had many interests, including mountain climbing, skiing, painting, playing the piano, and attending the theater, opera and concerts. As with many young ladies, she liked nice clothes, believing that simple beauty was becoming to a Christian lady. Concern for her neighbor was always a primary preoccupation with Gianna. She joined Catholic Action and participated in many of its charitable endeavors, especially visiting the poor and sick in their homes. She brought them food and medicines and tidied many a disorderly household.

When it came time to decide upon a life's work, Gianna decided upon medicine. She received her degree in medicine and surgery in 1949 from the University of Pavia in Italy. She then joined her brother, also a doctor, in his clinic in Mesero, located not far from the family home.

Gianna assisted many patients free of charge if they were too poor to afford medical help. She also supplied them with free medicine, supplies and money. Since she was especially attracted to serving mothers and children, she returned to school, while still maintaining her medical practice, and received a degree in pediatrics from the University of Milan in 1952. Gianna was a dedicated doctor who visited her patients in their homes in the countryside or in the hospital at Magenta. Sometimes she left her office as late as nine o'clock. She also promptly visited the sick at night.

Gianna seriously opposed abortion. She once wrote: "The doctor should not meddle. The right of the child to live is equal to the right of the mother's life . . . it is a sin to kill in the womb."

Still active in Catholic Action, Gianna met a mechanical engineer, Pietro Molla. After a seven-month engagement, Pietro, 43 years old, and Gianna, 33, were married by her brother, Father Giuseppe, in September of 1955. After an extended honeymoon touring Rome, the rest of Italy, and Europe, they settled in a little house near the plant where Pietro worked as director. Pietro wrote of his happiness with Gianna and agreed with her that they would form a truly Christian family, stating his hope that "we pray to be given the grace to be cheered by little angels."

Three months after the wedding, Gianna became pregnant,

and in due course, the couple's first child, Pier Luigi, was born. Then came Mariolina in 1957; then, two years later, Lauretta joined the family.

Serious complications had developed during each of the pregnancies. With all three Gianna had experienced excessive vomiting, intestinal binding and dysfunction and gastric disturbances that caused a great deal of pain. Her first pregnancy went 25 days beyond her due date, with labor of 36 hours. In the second pregnancy there were similar difficulties. The event was delayed ten days and was accompanied by a long and painful delivery. During the third pregnancy, Gianna had to be admitted to the hospital due to acute symptoms similar to those of her first two pregnancies. She suffered from vomiting and acute spasmodic contractions, accompanied by the threat of miscarriage. According to her obstetrician, the delivery of each child took place without pain relievers of any kind, in accord with the wishes of the mother.

In spite of the difficulties experienced, the births were immediate occasions for thankfulness and joy. After Baptism, each child was placed under the protection of Our Lady of Good Counsel, and as soon as she could, Gianna returned to her medical practice.

Gianna and Pietro prayed for yet another child to grace their family, but the next two pregnancies ended in spontaneous miscarriages. When Gianna became aware that she was again expecting, she soon realized that she was facing a serious, life-threatening experience. During her second month it was discovered that a painful fibroid tumor had grown in her uterus. Although a benign tumor, it was growing rapidly and threatened to compress the unborn child, bringing danger of abnormal development or miscarriage. Other complications also threatened, including a pre-term labor and displacement of the uterus.

There was also the possibility that the tumor might outgrow its blood supply and degenerate, causing considerable pain, as well as presenting the risk of infection.

Gianna, being a doctor, knew her options. The first was to have a hysterectomy, which would indirectly cause the death of the fetus and would preclude the possibility of future pregnancies. The second option would be to have the tumor removed, abort the fetus, but still retain the possibility of future pregnancies. These two options were not considered by Gianna since they would result in the death of the fetus. The third option was to have the tumor removed and continue the pregnancy, but this would present other serious complications. Gianna decided upon the third option.

The tumor was removed, and this pregnancy, like the others, was accompanied by nagging nausea and always the threat of a miscarriage. Gianna had suffered much during her other pregnancies, and without complaint. This last pregnancy, however, involved difficulties not faced in the previous ones, since the expanding uterus could press against the partially healed incision, breaking it open and causing a bloody hemorrhage.

Gianna remembered a lecture she once gave to the young girls of Catholic Action: "When the mother and child are in danger, the life of the child should take preference." When Gianna was given the same option, she immediately chose the life of the baby at a risk to her own. She was to say, "With faith and hope I am trusting in the Lord, even against science's terrible sentence. I trust in God, but now it is up to me to fulfill my duty as a mother. I renew the offering of my life to the Lord. I am ready for anything they will do to me, provided my child is saved."

After the fifth month, Gianna felt certain that the pregnancy would continue normally. She is said to have lived always calm and in apparent peace; and when she felt well enough, she returned to her patients until it was time for the birth.

On Good Friday of 1962, Gianna was admitted to the hospital, where labor was induced, but contractions were not forthcoming. It was then decided to deliver the baby by caesarean section. Under an ether anaesthetic, a healthy baby girl weighing almost ten pounds was delivered. She was named Gianna Emanuela.

A few hours later, Gianna's condition began to deteriorate. She experienced an elevated fever, a rapid and weakened pulse, and exhaustion. She also suffered an intense and overwhelming pain that was caused by septic peritonitis, an infection of the lining of the abdomen. Despite the extensive use of antibiotics, this condition was to continue for a week, until her death. During this painful abdominal suffering, Gianna declined all narcotic medications, since she wanted to remain perfectly awake. While suffering, she was heard to whisper frequently, "Jesus, I love You. Jesus, I love You!" Because of nausea she was unable to receive Holy Communion. Instead, the Sacred Host was placed on her lips.

Gianna knew she was dying, and she remarked to her sister, "If you only knew how differently things are judged at the hour of death; how vain certain things appear to which we give such importance in the world."

One week after the delivery, Gianna was taken home. Knowing she would soon die, she must have experienced an agony at the prospect of leaving her children, her dear husband, and the infant who needed the nurturing of its mother. Gianna is truly the model of a heroic mother who, for the life of her unborn child, sacrificed her own life, leaving in God's hands all those she loved in the world. Her doctor once exclaimed, "Behold the Catholic mother!"

Gianna died a few hours following her arrival home. It was

eight o'clock in the morning, the Saturday after Easter, April 28, 1962. Pietro was heartbroken at the loss of his beloved wife after only six and a half years of a happy married life. Two years later he was to suffer another tragedy when his oldest daughter, Mariolina, died.

Pier Luigi, Pietro Molla's only son, eventually entered the business world, married and raised a family, while Lauretta studied economics. Gianna Emanuela, who had been named for her mother, became a medical doctor and now cares for Alzheimer patients. She lives with her father in Magenta.

When Pope John Paul II conducted the beatification ceremony of Gianna Beretta Molla on April 24, 1994, in attendance were Gianna's husband, her surviving children and four of her sisters and brothers, all of whom received Holy Communion from the Pope. The feast day of Gianna was set for April 28, the anniversary of her entrance into eternal life.

Ten years later, on May 16, 2004, the Pope canonized Gianna. In attendance were her husband, her children and other family members. They witnessed the elevation of their beloved Gianna to the honors of the altar as a Saint of the universal Church.

39. SAINT GORGONIA (d. c. 375)

ORGONIA was born into a family of saints. She was the daughter of St. Gregory Nazianzen the Elder and St. Nonna, and she was the sister of the great St. Gregory Nazianzen, a Bishop and Doctor of the Church. She was married, the mother of three, and was known for her goodness and exemplary qualities. What we know of her is given by her brother, St. Gregory Nazianzen, during his funeral oration for his sister. Her many virtues were extolled, and then he related a tragedy that had befallen her:

"Her maddened mules ran away with her carriage, and unfortunately, overturned it; how horribly she was dragged along and seriously injured, to the shock of unbelievers . . . all crushed and bruised as she was, in bones and limbs, alike in those exposed and in those out of sight, she would have none of any physician to touch her, so that she owed her preservation to none other than to Him whom she loved and adored."

St. Gregory states that as a result of the accident, Gorgonia was left "with broken bones and crushed internal organs." Somehow she survived. Sometime later she suffered other afflictions, as described by her saintly brother: "She was sick in body and dangerously ill of an extraordinary and malignant disease; her whole frame was incessantly fevered, her blood at one time agitated and boiling, then curdling—with coma, incredible pallor, and paralysis of mind and limbs, and this not at long intervals, but sometimes very frequently. Its violence seemed beyond all human aid; the skill of physicians, who carefully examined the case, both singly and in consultation, was of no avail. What did the suffering soul do under these conditions? Despairing of all other aid, she betook herself to the Physician of all."

The Saint suffered for a time before surrendering her soul to God in full compliance with His holy Will.

Venerable Alberto
Capellan Zuazo
(p. 3)

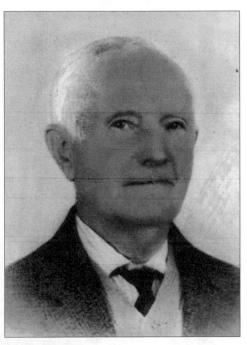

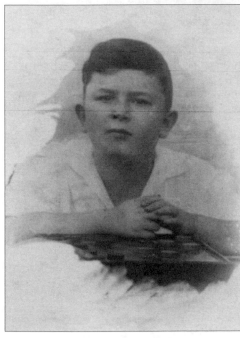

Servant of God
Aldo Blundo
(p. 6)

A

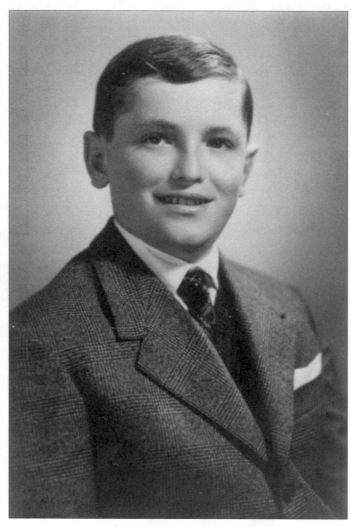

Servant of God Angiolino Bonetta (p. 30)

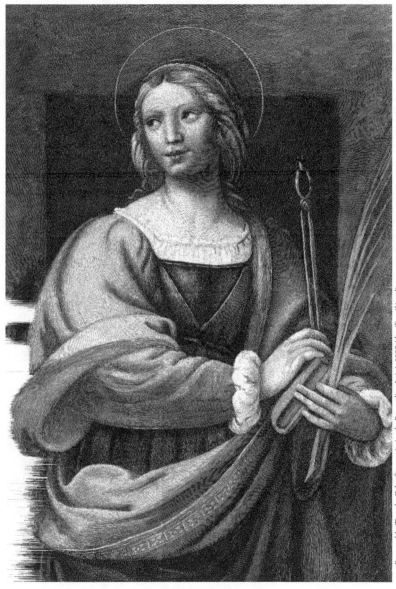

Saint Apollonia (p. 51)

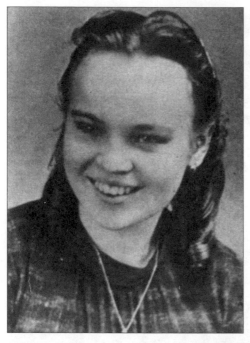

Servant of God
Annie Zelikova
(p. 44)

Venerable Antonietta
(Nennolina) Meo
(p. 47)

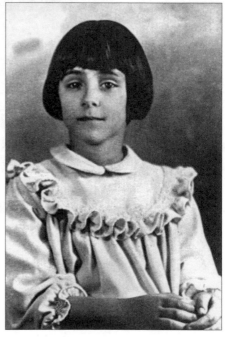

D

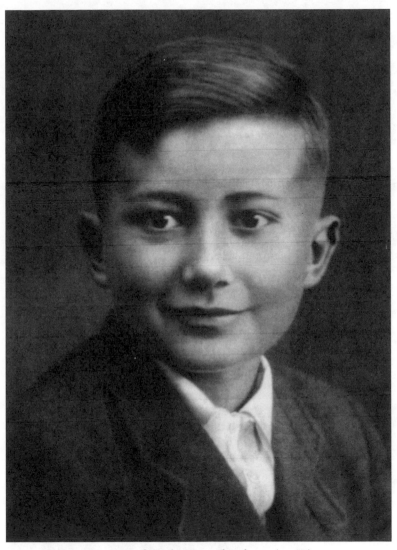

Servant of God Bernard Lehner (p. 55)

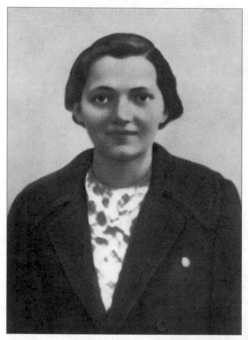

Servant of God
Angelina Pirini
(p. 28)

Venerable
Concepta Bertoli
(p. 70)

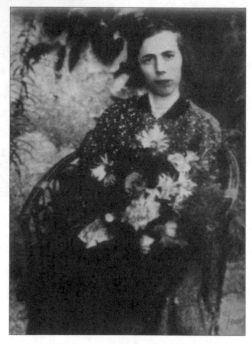

F

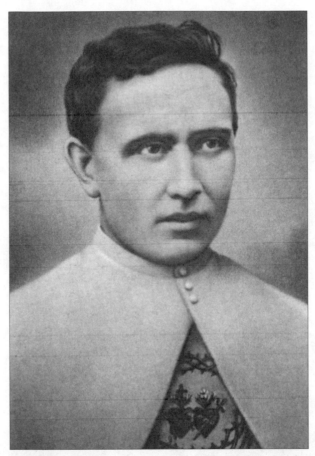

Saint Damien Joseph de Veuster of Molokai (p. 72)

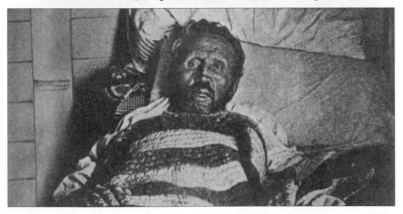

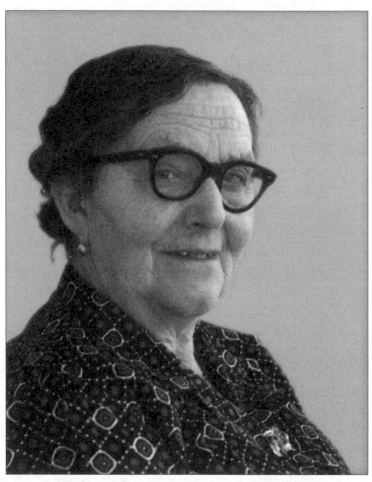

Servant of God Elisabetta Tasca Serena (p. 76)

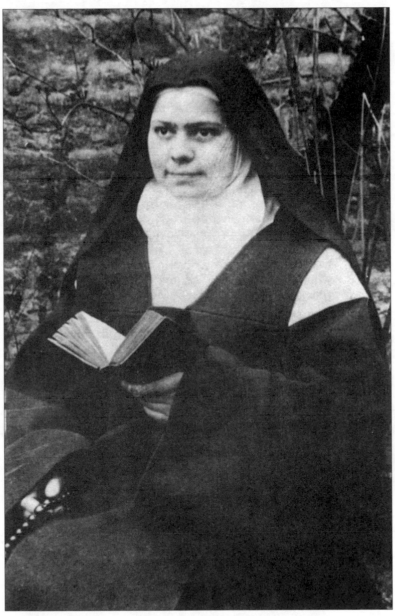

Blessed Elizabeth of the Trinity (p. 79)

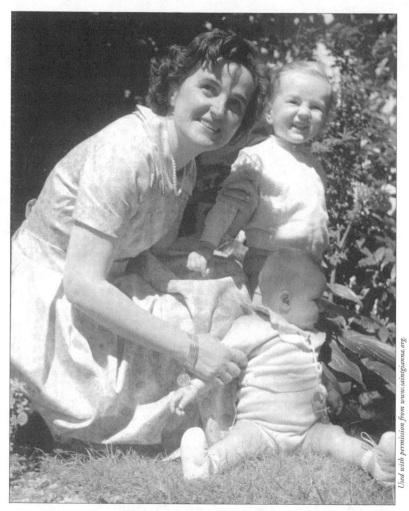

Saint Gianna Beretta Molla (p. 91) with her children

Servant of God
Faustino Perez-
Manglano (p. 81)

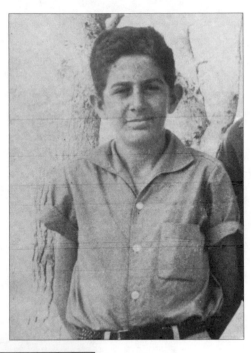

Venerable
Hildegard Burjan
(p. 107)

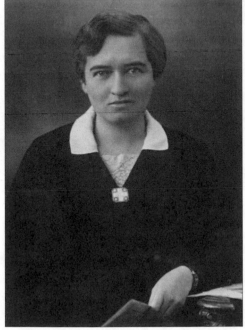

© Caritas Socialis

K

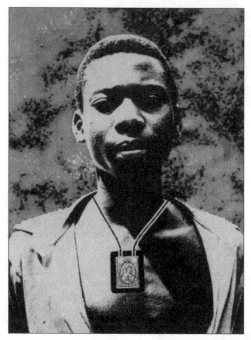

Blessed
Isidore Bakanja
(p. 111)

Servant of God
Luigi Rocchi
(p. 139)

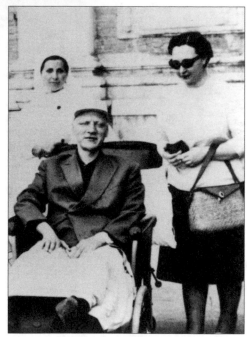

L

Venerable
Mari Carmen
Gonzalez-Valerio
(p. 154)

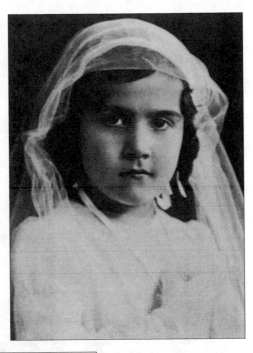

Servant of God
Maria Cristina Ogier
(p. 168)

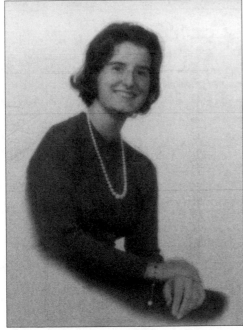

M

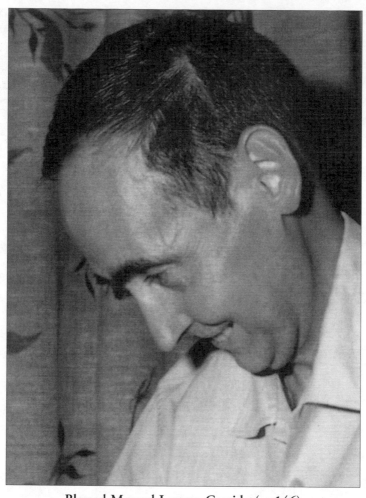

Blessed Manuel Lozano Garrido (p. 146)

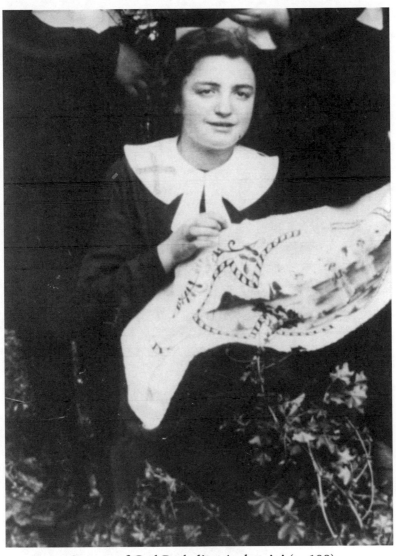

Servant of God Rachelina Ambrosini (p. 198)

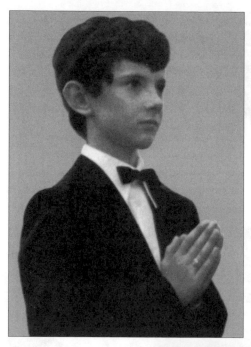

Servant of God
Silvio Dissegna
(p. 215)

Venerable
Stephen Kaszap
(p. 218)

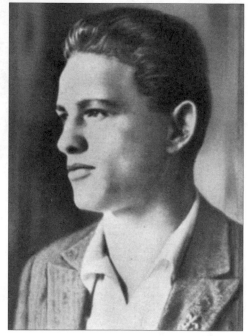

P

40. SAINT GREGORY THE GREAT
(540-604)

A MEMBER of a renowned senatorial family, Gregory the Great was born about the year 540. His mother, Sylvia, is venerated as a saint, as are two of his father's sisters, Tarsilla and Aemilia. Gregory received the best liberal education available at the time, but he considered that his spiritual and mental development came from his deeply religious family.

Because of his quick mind and organizational abilities, he attained the highest civil office in Rome by the time he was 30 years old and therefore wielded great authority in the city. Upon the death of his father, he became one of Rome's wealthiest men. With his inheritance he founded seven monasteries and converted his own home into the Monastery of St. Andrew, which he entered himself as a simple monk. But he was to spend only a few years in the monastic life—years which he subsequently proclaimed to have been the happiest of his life. He became a deacon and abbot and then arose, office by office, until he attained the highest position in the Church, being elected Pope in 590.

In February of 590, a plague was ravaging the area of Rome. In April, Pope Gregory organized a great procession to the Basilica of the Blessed Virgin. Carried in the procession was a picture of Our Lady that had reputedly been painted by St. Luke the Evangelist. When the procession reached the mausoleum of Hadrian, St. Gregory and all the people saw the Archangel

Michael standing on its summit sheathing his sword. This famous vision signaled the ending of the plague.

Named after Pope Gregory are the "Gregorian Masses," 30 consecutive daily Masses offered for the relief of the Souls in Purgatory. This custom developed when a monk fell ill and confessed that he had hidden three gold coins, a deed which was strictly against the poverty practiced by the monks. After his death he was ostracized by his fellows but St. Gregory, having pity on him, ordered that exactly 30 Masses be offered for the repose of his soul. When the deceased monk appeared all radiant and happy to one of the monks, the days were counted since the Masses had begun. They numbered exactly 30. Ever since, Gregorian Masses have been offered for departed souls with the confidence that the soul will either experience great relief or will obtain release from Purgatory.

Pope St. Gregory the Great is also known for his writings, of which his *Dialogues* is probably the best known. During his pontificate he also wrote many other literary works and more than 800 letters.

The Pope is also remembered for having laid the groundwork of the Roman liturgy in both Mass and Office. It is reported that although he did not compose the prayers, he arranged the parts. He composed eight of the hymns used in the Divine Office and founded two schools of chant, to which his name is forever affixed.

Although Gregory had accepted the office of Pope unwillingly, since he yearned to return to the monastery, he nevertheless performed all the duties of the papacy in good spirits and with great diligence, though suffering greatly from stomach troubles. It is surmised that the saint had developed this condition from imprudent penitential eating habits during his years as a monk.

In addition, he also suffered from the gout. He once wrote: "Sometimes the pain is moderate, sometimes excessive, but it is never so moderate as to leave me nor so excessive as to kill me. Hence it happens that I am daily in death and daily snatched from death."

To a friend he wrote: "At one time the pain of the gout tortures me, at another I know not what fire spreads itself over all my body; and sometimes it happens that at the same time the burning struggles with the pain, and body and mind seem to be leaving me." Yet Gregory's mind remained clear, and none of these struggles impeded his care of the Church or caused him to be absent from liturgical functions.

Pope St. Gregory is the last of the great Doctors of the ancient Church and is recognized to rightly deserve the title of "the Great."

41. SERVANT OF GOD GUIDO (GUY) DE FONTGALLAND (1913-1925)

GUIDO was only 11 years old when he died, yet he displayed a sanctity far beyond his years. He had been born on December 30, 1913 in Paris, where he attended school and received a good religious formation. The real starting point of his rapid rise in sanctity was the reception of his First Holy Communion. He displayed a keen interest in the Holy Sacrifice of the Mass and received Holy Communion with the utmost affection and eagerness.

His father, on seeing how attentive the boy was at Mass, asked Guido how one should occupy oneself during this time. He replied, "During Holy Mass our single occupation is to follow it thoughtfully. It is enough to read with the priest the prayers that he recites at the altar." Guido seems to have done that and more, since he often appeared to experience contemplative prayer during Mass.

Guido contracted diphtheria in December of 1924, and he knew instinctively that he would die. He expressed this to his mother. He lingered on for a month or so and endured without complaint all the ravages and sufferings of that disease. Guido died on January 24, 1925, a month into his 12th year. His sanctity became so well-known that the cause for his beatification was introduced in 1941.

42. BLESSED HENRY OF TREVISO (d. 1315)

ALSO known as Henry of Bolzano, the town where he was born in Italy, Henry suffered during an impoverished childhood and was unable to attend school. He never learned to read or write. To support himself, he journeyed to Treviso, where he found work as a day laborer.

Henry was a very spiritual man. He gave to the poor whatever he could spare from his meager wages and never missed an opportunity to serve God or his fellow man. He heard Mass daily and received the Eucharist as frequently as was customary at the time. When not employed in physical labor, Bl. Henry spent his time in prayer.

While it was obvious that Henry's soul was endowed with the beauty of spiritual graces, his physical appearance was definitely unattractive. He was a thick-set little man with dark sunken eyes, a long nose and a crooked mouth. Adding to his unattractive appearance were the shabby clothes he wore. He was frequently mocked and ridiculed by both children and adults, but he was never heard to utter a word of complaint, even when severely provoked. He never seemed to resent the treatment he received, and many marveled at his serenity under stress and his friendliness with everyone he met.

A charitable citizen gave Henry a room in his house when Henry could no longer work. He shared with beggars the food he was given and the alms he received from neighbors. It is said that he held over nothing from one day to the next.

Even after Henry was suffering from advanced age and bodily weakness, he continued to visit neighboring churches until the time of his death on June 10, 1315.

When Henry's death was announced, his little room was thronged with visitors who regarded him as a saint. Many of those who proclaimed his sanctity were persons who had formerly ridiculed his appearance. These and countless others were immediately scrambling for relics.

Miracles were soon reported, so that within a few days of his death, no fewer than 276 miracles were recorded. When the number increased, the magistrates of the town appointed notaries to keep a record of them. These miracles were reported by the Bollandists in the *Acta Sanctorum—The Acts of the Saints*. A biography of Bl. Henry of Treviso was written by his contemporary, Bishop Pier-Domenico de Baone. Bl. Henry, who had been mocked on earth for his unattractive appearance, is undoubtedly standing tall and handsome in the Kingdom of Heaven.

43. BLESSED HERMANN JOSEPH (d. 1241)

E ARE fortunate in that we have detailed information on the life of Blessed Hermann from a biography written by a contemporary. We are told that among the German mystics, Bl. Hermann proves to be of special interest, not so much for his writings as for his visions, which were a source of inspiration for many. Beginning with his early years in Cologne, Germany, the city of his birth, he was favored with frequent apparitions and conversations with Our Lady, the Child Jesus and the Angels. And he continued to be blessed with these visitations until his death in the year 1241.

After studying at the Premonstratensian monastery at Friesland, Bl. Hermann was professed and served the brethren for a time in the refectory. Later he was made sacristan, a position in which he delighted, since it gave him more time for prayer. The year of his Ordination is unknown, but what is recorded are the many ecstasies he experienced during the Holy Sacrifice of the Mass, at which he remained so long as to make many unwilling to act as servers.

Bl. Hermann proved to be a clever mechanic, especially in the repair of clocks. He is known to have composed prayers, hymns, two mystical treatises and other works which are said to have been inspired by Our Lady. Due to his excessive fasts and austerities, he endured severe headaches, which attacked him especially on the eve of great festivals. He endured these for many years until he was given a reprieve by Our Lord, who prolonged his life for another nine years. Bl. Hermann died of a fever and was buried at Hoven, but his incorrupt body was later translated to Steinfeld. Although his canonization process was never completed, his cultus was approved by the Vatican.

44. Venerable Hildegard Burjan
(1883-1933)

ILDEGARD Burjan was born in Goerlitz, Austria, of non-practicing Jewish parents. Little is known of her early years, but she is said to have been very intelligent, since at the age of 20 she was one of the first women to study philosophy in Zurich. There she met the Jewish engineer, Alexander Burjan. Two years later they were married, after which she completed her education and received her doctorate in philosophy.

Only one year after her marriage, Hildegard was struck with a serious problem involving her kidneys from which she almost died. This condition required four serious operations that produced such pain that only morphine gave her a little relief. She was blessed in being cared for in a hospital with Catholic nuns, for her survival and improvement were attributed to their prayers.

During her stay in the hospital, she observed the devoted care given to the patients by the Catholic nuns, and she began to learn about the Catholic Faith. She was eventually baptized, and at the age of 26 she envisioned leading a life of dedicated public service in co-operation with God's grace.

Hildegard moved to Vienna because of her husband's business, and it was there that she soon became pregnant. But then another serious kidney condition developed, and the doctors suggested that she abort the baby. Because of the strain of the pregnancy on her system, Hildegard's life was once more in danger, but she refused to submit to an abortion, calling it "murder." She told her physicians that she would rather risk her life for the sake of the child and that she would trust in God and in prayer. She eventually gave birth to a healthy daughter, whom she named Lisa.

Hildegard was fully aware of the social miseries in Vienna at that time, with children and young girls in danger, and rampant exploitation of female workers. To alleviate these and other problems, Hildegard began a Catholic women's organization known as *Caritas Socialis,* which effected a tremendous change. The organization established homes for the homeless, distributed food for the sick and the poor, and organized sewing rooms for unemployed women. With ten women who expressed a willingness to help, *Caritas Socialis* started an employment agency, convalescent homes, a hospital for the sick and insane, classes in various skills, and homes for unmarried mothers with children.

During all these charitable endeavors, Hildegard was still experiencing pain and various kidney difficulties, yet she somehow managed, without complaint, to continue with her work. In addition, she maintained a deep spiritual life, once commenting, "We must be completely filled by the insight that we can do nothing at all without grace." She also said, "I want to exhaust myself in love for others . . . Place all your concerns on God."

Hildegard suffered most of her life from kidney problems, which eventually became so severe that they claimed her life when she was 50 years old. The workers of *Caritas Socialis,* who continue the services that Hildegard initiated for the needy during her lifetime, continue this beautiful work in the memory of their foundress.

The cause for Hildegard's beatification was introduced in 1982. Her life of charity was declared one of heroic virtue in 2007.

45. Saint Ignatius of Loyola (1491-1556)

IGNATIUS was the last of 13 children and was born in the Basque country of Spain. His family belonged to the provincial nobility, and he served in the court of a relative during his youth. There he learned to gamble, to duel, and to perform with precision all of the court rituals. Ignatius entered the army in 1517 and fought in the battle of Pamplona in May of 1521. During the skirmish he received a serious leg wound that was to leave him with a permanent limp. While convalescing at his parents' villa at Loyola, he abandoned his worldly ways after reading the Life of Christ and the lives of the Saints. He had read these books because there was no worldly reading material available at the time.

Soon after his conversion, Ignatius had to struggle through a period of scrupulosity, during which he was tempted to despair of ever being worthy in God's sight. This was followed by a depression so severe that he actually considered suicide. We are told this by the Saint himself in his autobiography. Ignatius discovered that depression can be a great spiritual challenge and also a great opportunity for practicing virtue.

Ignatius, of course, persevered, so that he was favored with a vision of the Blessed Mother with the Child Jesus and was given a gift that he called the "Discretion of Spirits," a gift or spiritual power whereby he could distinguish between being inspired by God and being led in the wrong direction by other influences.

Ignatius eventually gave away his rich garments and assumed the clothing of a beggar. For the next ten months, he lived in a cave, where he received mystical graces and began writing the famed *Spiritual Exercises* that have served as the basis of countless retreats since 1535.

At the age of 33, he began university studies that would result in his receiving a Master of Arts degree from the University of Paris, having previously studied at Alcala and Salamanca. Eventually, his virtuous life caught the attention of several young men, including St. Francis Xavier, who wanted to follow his example. The result was the founding of the Society of Jesus, a religious Order otherwise known as the Jesuits.

Ignatius was ordained in 1537, and by 1540 the Order had received the approval of Pope Paul III. About this time, St. Francis Xavier began his journeys to the Far East as the first Jesuit missionary. The Jesuits began founding colleges and universities in 1542, and in 1543 the Saint organized several institutions for social outcasts.

Ignatius died in Rome on July 31, 1556 with the words, "Jesus, Jesus" on his lips. The Jesuits spread rapidly and have enriched the Church with 31 canonized Saints and 134 Beati.

46. Blessed Isidore Bakanja (1890-1904)

WHEN Belgian companies took possession of the Congo in Africa, they were intent on multiplying profits at the expense of the hard-working natives. The Trappists of Westmalle, Belgium were sent by Pope Leo XIII to help ease the inhumane treatment of the workers who labored in the rubber and ivory industries.

Isidore Bakanja was born around the time the Belgians arrived, and by his early teens he was in Mbandaka, where he obtained work as an assistant stonemason. Inspired by the missionaries, he was baptized and trained as a catechist. At the time of his Baptism, he was also enrolled in the Scapular Confraternity. From then on he was always seen wearing the Brown Scapular and reciting the Rosary.

After returning to his native village and his Boangi tribe, Isidore began to build a house for himself, and he accepted work as a servant boy. He became concerned that the Catholic Faith had not been preached in his region, and he began to instruct all who would listen to him. He eventually moved to Ikili, where he came to the attention of a violent, anti-Christian man named Van Cauter, who was also known as Longange. This anti-Christian ordered Isidore to stop teaching the natives, to stop praying the Rosary and to stop wearing the Scapular. A day later, as Isidore quietly continued his activities, Longange flew into a rage and ordered that Isidore be beaten with 25 strokes.

Another time, when Isidore was again found with the Scapular and the Rosary, Longange had two servant boys hold him down while he was beaten with a whip made of elephant hide that had two nails at one end which protruded through the hide. The boy was beaten between 200 and 250 times, with the nails tearing into the skin of his back. Afterward, when he rose from a pool of blood, he murmured, "The white man has killed me with his whip . . . He did not want me to pray to God. It is because I was praying to God."

Longange had Isidore chained by the feet in a room where rubber was processed, hoping the boy would die in isolation and that he would not be accused of the death. This began Isidore's Calvary, since he was deposited on a dirty mat in a filthy room where mosquitos and insects tormented his infected wounds and where the dense odor of burning rubber caused him severe coughing spells.

Isidore was discovered by an inspector, who promptly disciplined Longange. The inspector had Isidore brought to his boat, where he personally tended the wounds. A young servant boy remembers: " . . . I slept near him, Isidore on the bed and I by the fire in front of the bed. Isidore had been terribly wounded, but he never abandoned his prayers. He prayed very much . . . "

The serious condition of Isidore was too much for his caregivers, so he was moved from place to place, but eventually he spent his last days living on the porch of a catechist. Father Gregoire visited him often and heard his Confession and anointed him on July 24, 1909. Isidore also received the Holy Eucharist, much to his joy and consolation. He told Fr. Gregoire, "It's nothing if I die. If God wants me to live, I'll live! If God wants me to die, I'll die. It is all the same to me." And then, in spite of the pain caused by his terribly infected wounds, he added, "I'm not angry with the white man. He beat me. That is his business; it is none of mine. He should know what he is doing . . . I shall pray for him when I am in Heaven. I shall pray for him very much."

Isidore's wounds were dressed with medicines provided by the director of the Belgian company, but the wounds were too infected to hope for a cure. In time, Isidore's whole body became infected, with his hips and bones protruding through his skin. His neck also caused atrocious pains from the kicks he had received from Longange the day of his beating. Throughout this ordeal, Isidore was often seen praying his Rosary.

Eventually, on Sunday, August 8, Isidore began vomiting blood and decaying matter. All this time he was forced to lie on his stomach because of his festering wounds. In this position every movement caused additional pain.

The next Sunday, Isidore somehow participated in the prayers held by the Catholics. He ate a simple meal, returned to his mat and died peacefully. He was only 14 years old.

The Congo, now known as Zaire, won its independence from Belgium in 1960. When Pope John Paul II visited the country 20 years later, in 1980, he praised Isidore Bakanja, stating that Isidore was "a true Christian. After having given all his free time to the evangelization of his brothers as a catechist, he did not hesitate to offer his life to God, strong in the courage he found in his faith and in the faithful recitation of the Rosary."

Since Isidore had been inscribed in the registry of the parish Confraternity of the Scapular at his Baptism, the Council of the Carmelite Order in 1984 declared that Isidore was a "gift from God and from the Blessed Virgin Mary. The Scapular devotion has its martyr." Isidore was beatified by the Pope on April 24, 1994.

47. Servant of God Isidoro Zorzano
(1902-1943)

ISIDORO was born in Buenos Aires, Argentina, but his family relocated to Spain when Isidoro was only three. He excelled in his school studies and eventually obtained a degree in industrial engineering.

When Isidoro was 28 years old he decided that one need not abandon the world in order to be holy, since ordinary work could become a means of holiness and service to the Church. Isidoro realized that his desire to seek higher spirituality while continuing his profession could be realized. From that day forward, he dedicated himself completely to God. In the midst of his many occupations he daily devoted a half hour to mental prayer in the morning and again in the afternoon. He also attended daily Mass and received Holy Communion, and he was faithful in the evening to the daily examination of faults.

During the Spanish Civil War of 1936-1939, which produced great persecution for the Church, many Catholics went into hiding or moved to other places. A group of revolutionaries had already sentenced Isidoro to death for his many religious activities, forcing him to leave his position with the Andalusian Railway. When the war ended in 1939 and peace was restored, Isidoro returned to his former occupation.

When Isidoro was almost 41, his health began to decline. In the hospital his condition was diagnosed as Hodgkin's disease, a malignant, progressive, sometimes fatal disease that causes enlargement of lymph nodes and other organs. He endured great suffering for six months and was administered the Sacrament of Anointing of the Sick. Isidoro passed to his eternal reward in 1943 on the eve of the feast of Our Lady of Mount Carmel, that is, on July 15. He was buried the next day in the Almudena Cemetery in Madrid.

Five years later, after so many answers to prayer through his intercession had been reported, the informative process for beatification was started. It was concluded on June 17, 1994. Isidoro is now known as a Servant of God.

48. Blessed James Alberione
(1884-1971)

HIS devout farming family in northern Italy encouraged and supported Giacomo—James—when he felt called to the priesthood. At the age of 17, he entered the seminary in Alba, Italy. He was engaged in a four-hour Eucharistic adoration during the night when the century changed from 1900 to January 1, 1901. It was then that he felt inspired to serve the people of the 20th century in a new, creative way.

This thought lingered with James after his ordination in June of 1907. But first, he was obliged to serve as the parish priest in Narzole. Then, while serving as spiritual director for youth in the Alba seminary, he decided to both teach the boys a trade and also help the Church at the same time by printing a weekly paper called the *Gazzetta d'Alba,* which was inaugurated in September of 1913. The success of his endeavor to advance the boys in the spiritual life while performing this work can be gauged by one of these young boys, Venerable Maggiorino Vigolungo (d. 1918), who is now a candidate for canonization. (His story is told in this book.)

The following year, Fr. James Alberione founded the Society of St. Paul. A year later he founded the Daughters of St. Paul. In addition to these two religious organizations, Fr. James founded a number of others, including the Pious Disciples of the Divine Master, the Sisters of the Queen of the Apostles, the Secular Institute of St. Gabriel, the Annunciationist Institute,

116

the Holy Family Institute for married people, and the Institute of Jesus the Priest for the secular clergy. These organizations were so successful in obtaining vocations that as a result, priests, brothers and sisters were sent to over 30 countries.

Fr. James was aware of the changes in world culture and the evil that was beginning to be spread through the press, and he believed that technology had to be used to counteract it. Thus it is that the work of the Pauline family uses books, magazines, computer technologies and television to advance the spread of Christian ideals to people who rarely visit churches for religious instruction.

With all that this holy priest accomplished, it is hard to believe that he always had limited energies and was frequently ailing. When he was in his 40s and already busy with his fast-growing communities, he was diagnosed with a terminal case of tuberculosis. He suffered with this until, as he revealed, he was cured by St. Paul. No particulars of this cure were ever given, he being reticent to divulge anything in his life that would detract from the attention due to God.

The holy priest lived another 40 years after the spectacular cure, but other physical difficulties arose. What was particularly troublesome was the region of his upper spine, the thoracic region, which was extremely curved and which could be identified as manifesting a condition known as scoliosis. Modern doctors might diagnosis it as such, but a definitive determination was never made. The good priest also suffered excruciatingly from arthritis in the spinal region, so that he was barely able to sleep but four hours a night. Despite this, he maintained a schedule of activities which began with Holy Mass at 4 o'clock in the morning.

After a full life of accomplishments for the Church, Fr. James Alberione died at the age of 89 in the generalate house in Rome on November 26, 1971. He was beatified by Pope John Paul II on April 27, 2003. His numerous religious organizations anxiously await the canonization of their founder, Blessed James Alberione.

49. SAINT JANE OF VALOIS (1464-1505)

JANE'S parents were King Louis XI of France and Charlotte of Savoy. She was a disappointment and an object of aversion to her father because of her small stature and misshaped body, due to a severe deformity of her spine. As was the custom of the time, her father betrothed her to a cousin, Louis, Duke of Orleans, when she was only a child. When Jane's future mother-in-law met her for the first time a few years later, she vowed to break the engagement. But the King responded by threatening the life of the intended bridegroom. The marriage eventually took place when Jane was only 12 years old.

When her husband was accused of rebellion, Jane was successful in saving his life by pleading with her brother, Charles VIII, who had become King of France. In spite of this, nothing could conquer his dislike of her. When the unwilling husband came to the throne as Louis XII, he sent envoys to Rome to obtain a declaration of nullity ("annulment") of his marriage to Jane, chiefly on the grounds that she had been forced upon him by Louis XI. After carefully studying the matter based on witness testimonies, Pope Alexander VI agreed, and the marriage was declared invalid. Louis XII then advantageously married Anne, the heiress of Brittany and the late King's widow.

Since Jane offered no opposition to the declaration of nullity, Louis XII, in appreciation, gave her various properties. She lived at Bourges, devoting herself to mortification, prayer and works of charity. In the year 1500 she founded an Order of nuns dedicated to the Annunciation of the Blessed Virgin, an Order also

119

known as the Franciscan Annunciades of Bourges, which has been approved by four Popes. St. Jane received the habit three years later and died the following year, after suffering throughout her life from the pains caused by her deformity.

50. SAINT JOHN OF GOD (d. 1550)

OHN was born in Portugal of parents who were good and pious, but poor. For most of his childhood he worked as a shepherd, and then in 1522, he enlisted in a company of foot soldiers and served in various battles in both Spain and Hungary. He followed the licentious behavior of his companions and gradually lost his piety and ceased his practices of religion. When the troop was disbanded, he returned to his work as a shepherd and thus had time to consider his past misconduct. He then resolved to amend his life and do penance for his sins. At this time John was about 40 years old. He then realized that by turning peddler, and selling little sacred pictures and devotional books, he would not only help his customers, but he would also make a little money with which to help the poor. He did so well in this regard with one shop that he opened another one in Granada.

When the servant of God, John of Avila, who was known as the Apostle of Andalusia, came to the city on a special invitation to preach, John attended the sermon. He was so greatly affected and so sorry for his sins that he began to cry aloud in church for God's mercy. He began beating his breast and then ran about the streets, pulling out his hair, tearing his clothes and throwing himself into puddles of mud while publicly confessing his sins. He behaved so wildly that he was pelted with stones by children, who called him a madman. At one point John returned to his shop, gave away his stock and began tearing the pages of books with his teeth.

He was brought before John of Avila, who quieted him by

telling him to forgo his mortifications, which had reduced him to a weakened state. He gave John proper advice and heard his Confession. John was quieted for a time, but then he began again to run through the streets, shouting for God's mercy.

Finally, two citizens had pity on him and took him by the hand and led him through the crowd to the Royal Hospital, where the insane of the city received treatment, although in those days the treatment was harsh and cruel. After a time John recovered and was released. Determined to help the poor, he began to collect wood, which he then sold, distributing the money among the poor and the sick. He rented a house, where he served the sick with such charity that the whole city was astonished. Eventually, John's charity was recognized by the Bishop of Tuy and members of the nobility, who donated monies for the relief of those he tended.

In time, John attracted followers, who were given a habit by the Bishop. After John's death, a Rule was drawn up and religious vows were introduced.

John is recognized for a miracle that took place when his little foundation for the sick was enveloped in flames. John went back into the establishment time and time again, bringing the sick to safety. It was noted as a miracle that he passed through the flames without injury.

The Saint died on March 8, 1550 at the age of 55. His funeral was conducted by the Archbishop before countless priests, the nobility and the whole of Granada. Many miracles were obtained through his intercession, and he was canonized by Alexander VIII in 1690. Pope Leo XIII declared St. John of God to be the "heavenly patron of all hospitals and the sick." He is also honored as the patron of printers and booksellers.

The Order that he started is known as the Brothers Hospitallers of St. John of God, or simply as the Hospitallers.

51. Saint Josemaria Escriva
(1902-1975)

JOSEMARIA was one of six children born to Jose and Dolores Escriva in Barbastro, Spain. When the young boy was 12 years old the family moved to Logrono for economic reasons. In the last days of 1917 Josemaria realized a first calling to the priesthood when he saw footprints left in the snow by a passing monk. He studied in both Logrono and Zaragoza and was ordained in the latter on March 28, 1925. After serving as a parish priest, he moved to Madrid in 1927 to study law. Two years later we find him creating for lay people an organization known as Opus Dei (Latin for "God's Work"). Through this movement Josemaria meant to help Catholics learn that sanctity can be achieved without abandoning the secular life.

During the infamous Spanish Civil War of 1936-1939, Josemaria went into hiding to escape persecution by anti-clerics, yet he continued to risk his life in order to minister to faithful Catholics. When hostilities ended, he resumed his studies for a doctorate in law and was often invited by bishops to preach spiritual retreats to the clergy. Another organization founded by the holy priest was the Priestly Society of the Holy Cross, begun in the year 1943.

Josemaria moved to Rome in 1946 and obtained his doctorate in theology. Pope Pius XII acknowledged Escriva's work by granting Opus Dei his official approval on June 16, 1950. The Pope also honored him by appointing him Consultor to two Vatican Congregations, and he was made an honorary member of the Pontifical Academy of Theology.

About this time Josemaria had already been suffering for ten years from serious diabetes, but we are told that he was miraculously cured and that, with the restoration of his health, he continued to encourage membership in Opus Dei throughout Spain, Portugal, Mexico and South America. By the time of his death, Opus Dei was known on five continents, with a membership of 60,000 members of 80 nationalities.

Josemaria wrote a number of spiritual works and was considered a saint before his death on June 26, 1975. His cause was introduced six years later, and he was canonized by Pope John Paul II on October 6, 2002.

During the canonization ceremony the Pope made the following observation: "With supernatural intuition, St. Josemaria untiringly preached the universal call to holiness and apostolate. Christ calls everyone to become holy in the realities of everyday life. Hence work too is a means of personal holiness and apostolate when it is done in union with Jesus Christ."

52. SAINT JULIANA FALCONIERI (1270-1341)

JULIANA was a member of a noble Florentine family and the niece of St. Alexis Falconieri, who was one of the seven founders of the Servite Order. From her earliest youth she consecrated herself to the religious life and the practice of Christian perfection. After her father's death, she received the habit of the Servite Third Order from St. Philip Benizi, her spiritual director and one of the founders of the Order. She lived at home observing the Rule until her mother's death in 1304, when she, with several companions, moved into a house which became the first convent of the Servite Third Order.

Juliana was elected as the first superior. She and her companions adopted a habit and devoted themselves especially to the care of the sick and to works of mercy. For 35 years Juliana directed the community, until a chronic gastric condition from which she had suffered since her youth made it impossible to continue.

We are told that her constant vomiting made it impossible for her to receive the Eucharist before her death. Instead, she asked the priest to spread a corporal upon her chest and lay the Sacred Host upon it. After the Host suddenly disappeared, Juliana died, but the image of the cross that had been on the Host was found on her breast. Juliana died on June 12, 1341. She is often portrayed in art wearing a full habit with a Host present on her chest.

Juliana was beatified in 1678 and was canonized on June 16, 1737 by Pope Clement XII. The Order of Servite Tertiaries was sanctioned by Pope Martin V in 1420.

53. Blessed Kateri Tekakwitha
(1656-1680)

ATERI was the daughter of a young Mohawk chief and a mother who had been converted to the Catholic Religion in Southeast Canada by French missionaries. When their tribe lived near the Mohawk River at a place known as Ossernenon, now known as Auriesville, New York, they became the parents of a beautiful daughter. Since it was felt that only a priest should perform Baptism, it was years before Kateri received this Sacrament.

The family was happy until the year 1660, when an epidemic of smallpox claimed a third of the Ossernenon population. Kateri's mother, father and younger brother all contracted the disease and died. Only Kateri, at four years of age, survived, but she would retain a reminder of the disease for the rest of her life in the form of badly pitted skin on her formerly beautiful face. As a result of the disease, she also developed a weakness of vision, with an extreme sensitivity to light. Bright sunshine or the glare of water or snow would be a source of pain to her throughout her life. All was well while she worked in the dim longhouse, but outside, if the weather was bright and clear, Kateri found it necessary to shield her eyes and grope her way to where she intended to go. She was finally given the name "Tekakwitha," which translates into "She-who-feels-her-way-along," or "She-who-pushes-with-her-hands."

After the death of her father, the little orphan was adopted by her uncle, the chief of the Turtle clan, who placed Kateri in the care of her aunts. Thereafter, these aunts schemed together and planned to have her married, hoping to provide the family with a young brave who would assist with the hard work, as well as with the hunting and fishing. Kateri had other plans. A few years earlier, when she was 11 years old, the village had been visited by three Jesuit missionaries. After listening to them and attending Catholic religious services, Kateri began to look forward to being a Catholic and leading a life of prayer. It is reported that when she refused to accept the marriage proposal of a young brave whom the aunts had selected for her, she voluntarily left the longhouse, although another biographer claims that she was expelled by her angered family.

Kateri's desire to become a Christian was confided to Fr. Jacques de Lamberville, who instructed her in the "wigwam of prayer" and baptized her on Easter Sunday, April 5, 1676, when she was 18 years old. It was then that she was given the name Kateri in honor of St. Catherine of Alexandria.

Kateri was now faced with persecution from her uncle, who resented her conversion, especially when she refused to work in the fields on Sundays. Her aunts accused her of idleness and refused to give her food on the days she did not work. Although Kateri already performed most of the housework, her aunts pressured her with commands throughout the day in an effort to break her will. Scoldings and mockery had proved successful with other converts, who had given in under the strain, but Kateri bore the persecution with humility and remained steadfast. She eventually moved, at the recommendation of the priests, to the Mission of St. Francis Xavier at Kahnawake, where she had complete freedom to express her faith and exercise her devotion. She pronounced vows and consecrated herself entirely to the Blessed Virgin.

During the last few years of her life, Kateri suffered from

headaches, a fever, painful stomach cramps, and frequent vomiting. This did not deter her from practicing various penances, which unfortunately greatly reduced her strength. As a result of these conditions, Kateri became very weak and was confined to bed. She received the Last Sacraments and quietly died at three o'clock in the afternoon on April 17, 1680. She was not quite 24 years old.

A miracle took place soon after her death: eyewitnesses saw the ravages of sickness disappear from Kateri's face, to give way to a fresh, smiling and radiant countenance. Even the pock marks that had disfigured her face from childhood could no longer be seen. Later, many testified to this marvel under oath.

Kateri's remains are kept in a marble sarcophagus in the Church of St. Francis Xavier in Kahnawake, Quebec, which continues to be a place of devotion for thousands of pilgrims. Kateri was proclaimed Venerable in 1941 by Pope Pius XII and was beatified on June 22, 1980 by Pope John Paul II.

54. SERVANT OF GOD
LORENA D'ALEXANDER (1964-1981)

*L*ORENA was born in La Rustica, a district on the out-skirts of Rome, to a family of modest means. She was an intelligent and happy child, but of a delicate phys-ical nature. It seems as though she was destined for suffering, since at the age of 10 she had operations for both tonsillitis and appendicitis. That same year a malignant tumor was discovered in her left leg. An immediate operation was performed to remove the tumor and replace it with bone taken from another area of her body. All seemed to go well until after she received the Sacrament of Confirmation in 1976, when the tumor returned. The only means left to preserve her life was the ampu-tation of the leg. Lorena accepted the news as the Will of God and co-operated cheerfully with all the pre-operative tests and the post-operative remedies, and it was she who reassured her worried parents that all would be well.

Lorena was not one to lie in bed or to pity herself, and she was soon up and about in a wheelchair visiting other patients and telling them little stories to relieve their concerns. She was always welcomed by the sick, who found great comfort in her visits.

She was soon fitted with a prosthesis and began almost immediately to join the young people at her parish who were engaged in catechetical work. She was especially delighted when, in 1979, she was given her own class of youngsters. She fully realized that "happiness will always be in serving the happiness of others, in being of service to others."

Lorena studied at the high school named Pilo Albertelli in Rome, and she joined her friends in making a pilgrimage to Lourdes in August 1980. She bathed in the miraculous waters and wrote home to tell of her experiences. She mentioned that she was inspired by the suffering of so many who bore their pains in silent prayer.

Lorena had the great pleasure during the rest of 1980 of living with other catechists in a parish building. This experience contributed to her spiritual maturity and her rapid rise in sanctity. At this time she wrote, "I have understood that the most important thing is to live of love, to live for love, to live with love."

At the beginning of the year 1981 Lorena's happy life as a catechist was abruptly ended when it was discovered that the cancer had metastasized, with a tumor destroying her left lung. All who knew the devout teenager were devastated at the news, but she consoled them with a smile, saying, "Don't cry, but rejoice with me because if the good Lord thinks me worthy, I will join Him in glory. This will be the greatest joy of all."

The doctors declared that Lorena would live only three months, and she knew that to be true. Nevertheless, various painful remedies were attempted, to which Lorena submitted willingly and cheerfully. Despite the care she received and the attempts made to save her life, Lorena died on April 3, 1981 when she was only 16 years old.

Only 18 years later, on October 4, 1999, the cause for Lorena's beatification was introduced with the assignment of a postulator.

45. SAINT LOUIS IX, KING OF FRANCE
(1215-1270)

ST. LOUIS was crowned King of France at the age of 11, shortly after the death of his father, Louis VIII. His mother, Blanche of Castile, was responsible for forming the character of the young King and was particularly careful "to instill into his soul the highest regard and awe for everything that pertained to divine worship, religion and virtue." Unfortunately, when Louis, at the age of 19, married Margaret, the daughter of Raymond Berenger, Count of Provence, his mother became troublesome, due to her jealousy of her daughter-in-law. Despite the trouble she made for Margaret in trying to keep the husband and wife apart, Margaret and Louis were blessed with 11 children, five sons and six daughters.

Among Louis' many good traits was his outstanding generosity to the poor, giving liberally of what he had. He customarily waited upon the poor as they sat about his table and even cut the meat for those who were unable to do so. Each guest was also given coins before he left. St. Louis helped religious Orders, provided dowries for needy girls who wished to be married, sheltered many homeless women and established a house for them near Paris. He is also known to have visited hospitals, where he would perform the most menial services for the sick. He even went so far as to care for a greatly disfigured leper, patiently feeding him and performing other services for him.

Although the King often ministered to the sick, he was not a well man himself, yet he gave no evidence that his frail constitution ever prevented him from fulfilling any of his responsibilities. The main cause of his condition was the malarial infection he had contracted and from which he never entirely recovered. In addition, he suffered attacks of erysipelas (a feverish and acute disease often attacking the face, producing an intense reddish inflammation of the skin and underlying tissues).

Despite his physical ailments, the Saint participated in two crusades and was taken prisoner after the first one. During his imprisonment, he endured harshness, sickness, insults, frequent interrogations, and chains. As a result of the second crusade, Louis fell victim to the same disease that claimed many of his troops. He received the Last Sacraments and died on August 25, 1270.

Considered a saint during his lifetime, King Louis IX was canonized by Pope Boniface VIII in 1297. His feast day is observed on August 25, the anniversary of his death.

56. BLESSED LOUIS MARTIN (1823-1894)

*L*OUIS Martin, the father of St. Thérèse of the Child Jesus and of the Holy Face, was born at Bordeaux, France, one of four children, and was the son of an army captain. Given the name, Louis Joseph Aloys Stanislaus, he was baptized shortly after his birth. At the age of 19, Louis first went to Rennes to learn watchmaking and then was apprenticed in Strasbourg. While there, he visited the Augustinian Monastery of Mount St. Bernard, where he hoped to be admitted. He was turned away, being told to learn Latin and then return. Louis studied the language for a time, and then realized his vocation was in the secular world.

Louis established himself at Alencon as a master watchmaker and opened a shop that was enlarged to include jewelry. When he was 35 years old, he met and married Zelie Guerin in 1858, with whom he lived as brother and sister for ten months, until his spiritual director suggested that he consider the vocation of parenthood. Nine children were eventually born to the couple, but four of them died while very young. Eventually, Louis sold his business to his nephew and devoted his time and energy to Zelie's lace-making business, which thrived under his skill as a salesman and manager. After 19 years of marriage, Zelie Martin (see her entry in this book) died in 1877 of breast cancer at age 45, leaving her grieving husband to raise their five daughters: Marie, Pauline, Leonie, Celine and Thérèse, who ranged in ages from 17 to 4. Louis sold Zelie's lace-making business and moved to Lisieux with his daughters to be near his brother-in-law, Isidore Guerin, and Isidore's wife.

After three daughters entered the Discalced Carmelite Order and one the Visitation Order, it was Celine who stayed home to care for her father, who had suffered a paralytic stroke in 1887, temporarily affecting his left side. He recovered completely, but soon he began to suffer from arteriosclerosis and to experience delusions, amnesia and severe lapses of memory. He even began, on a number of occasions, to wander away from home. Monsieur Martin's Calvary had begun. Because the family feared for his safety, Louis Martin was placed in a mental hospital. There he was admired by the nursing sisters not only because of his daughters in religion, but also because he never complained but accepted every inconvenience as being the Will of God. He once admitted, "I know why God has given me this trial. I have never had a humiliation in my life. I needed one."

A year after the first stroke, he suffered another that paralyzed his legs. Since he was no longer able to wander away, he was permitted to return home. With the help of a married couple who were employed as servants, Celine was able to devote all her attention to her pious father—a loving service she rendered him for the next three years. On days when he was able, he enjoyed visiting his daughters in religion, who were so worried about his condition.

After a stroke that paralyzed his left arm, Louis suffered a series of heart attacks that weakened him and heralded the approach of death. With his body paralyzed, his speech impaired and his faculties reduced to helplessness, he begged the good Lord to take him home. After the last heart attack he received the Last Sacraments of the Church and died quietly on July 27, 1894. He was 71 years old. He had been in a pitiful state of illness for seven years.

After his death, Celine joined her three sisters in the Discalced Carmelite monastery. All the sisters were alive when Thérèse, who died at 24, was canonized by Pope Pius XI in 1925.

Louis Martin and his wife Zelie were both beatified on October 19, 2008 at the Basilica of Lisieux by José Cardinal Saraiva Martins, the legate of Pope Benedict XVI.

57. VENERABLE LOUIS NECCHI VILLA
(1876-1930)

*L*OUIS Necchi Villa was born in Italy. He is the only person in this book whose parents were divorced. Unable to support her children by herself after the divorce, his mother married Federico Villa, a sculptor.* The divorce of his parents, the subsequent upheaval in the family, and the introduction of his stepfather may well have been the sources of the neurosis from which Louis would suffer the rest of his life.

In spite of the atmosphere in the home that did not foster religion, Louis did receive his First Communion at the age of 12. He was enrolled in Parini High School, where one of his classmates was Edward Gemelli, the future Padre Agostino, with whom he was to have a lifelong friendship. Louis did not practice his religion during those years, but he experienced a conversion in 1893 at the age of 17.

After high school, he enrolled at the College Leo XIII, where he met Father Guido, who was to be his spiritual director for the next 30 years. Afterwards, he enrolled in the school of medicine at Pavia. In a scholastic environment hostile to religion, Louis became involved in debates on social problems in which he championed the ideas of the Christian's social duties according to papal teachings. He spoke of absolute fidelity to the teachings of the encyclical *Rerum Novarum,* and he worked for

---

* It would appear that this was only a civil union, not a valid marriage recognized by the Church.—*Publisher,* 2010.

the social progress of city workers and farmers.

Louis graduated with a degree in medicine in 1902 and briefly joined the military, where he worked in the military hospital of St. Ambrogio. When a friend entered the seminary, Louis wondered if he also was called to the priesthood and took a course of spiritual exercises. He concluded that he was called to the state of Matrimony and to the secular apostolate.

Louis practiced medicine in Berlin and found time to develop an apostolate for Italian emigrants to Germany. He also found time to court Victoria Della Silva, whom he married in Milan in 1905. Their union was blessed with three children.

Dr. Villa was asked three years later to join the diocesan committee of Catholic Works and soon became president of the group. He remained in that position for most of his life. He held other offices and again returned to a military hospital during World War I, where he worked for 18 months.

After Louis' return to civilian life, he began to do research in the mental aspects of psychology and biology, devoting himself to the care of the sick with nervous problems and of children with abnormal traits. Having himself experienced a mental disorder since childhood, he understood the problem and organized a department in the Institute St. Vincent for the education of children. He remained the department's director for ten years.

Dr. Villa's social and medical activities were many, as were the articles he wrote for various journals. He was helpful in the foundation of the Catholic University of the Sacred Heart, and he accepted the position of professor in the department of biology and a chair on the faculty of philosophy.

In the autumn of 1929, the doctor underwent several surgical procedures. The first operation revealed a malignant tumor from which he had suffered miserably, but which he had concealed behind a constant smile. Death claimed the holy doctor on January 10, 1930 at the age of 54.

Following his death, many biographies appeared, and many were translated into various languages. His body is now found in the chapel of the Catholic University of the Sacred Heart, where on his tombstone, in addition to his name and pertinent dates, are found the words, "Franciscan Tertiary."

One of the doctor's biographies states: "The life of this man, tormented by doubt and by neurosis, shows that this does not contrast with holiness. The weight of the psychic conditioning, which the Venerable sometimes experienced, under the action of the Holy Spirit can be approved and lived as a means of sanctification. Louis Necchi Villa knew how to love, to work and to produce benefits for the society in which he lived with inexhaustible fertility."

The cause for Louis' beatification was initiated by Cardinal Schuster three years after his death and was eventually introduced in 1951. He was elevated to the position of Venerable in 1971.

58. Servant of God Luigi Rocchi
(1932-1979)

*L*UIGI Rocchi was born in 1932 in Tolentino, Italy, the city made famous by St. Nicholas of Tolentino. He was healthy until the age of 19, when he began to experience the early signs of muscular dystrophy. His condition became progressively worse until, by the age of 28, his hands and feet were paralyzed, and he was completely immobile. His immobility lasted for 19 years, but this did not stop him from giving comfort to souls who suffered in mind or spirit.

From the earliest days of his sickness, he became so well known for his cheerfulness and optimistic attitude that many were attracted to him, so that he was always either receiving visitors or answering their letters. For a time he could write the letters, but when his hands became paralyzed, he beat the keys of a typewriter with a stick he held in his mouth. It is reported that he wrote as many as 22 letters in one day, and in these he gave comfort to other people and communicated his joy of living and his love of God and nature. Many of these letters have been preserved and have been reprinted in various publications.

All who met Luigi were struck by his great joy and by his love for everyone. When asked about the source of his gaiety, he replied: "What is the secret of my joy? I am thirsty for God. So much thirst for God."

Luigi's mother was his attentive and caring nurse. She once confided that in the beginning of her nursing duties, she had experienced great difficulty, but because of Luigi's cheerfulness and prayerful attitude, she found her chores much more agreeable and less tiring. In fact, even though Luigi suffered a great deal, he accepted his condition in imitation of the crucified Jesus and never complained.

One of his admirers was Monsignor Capovilla, the secretary of Pope John XXIII, who wrote, "Luigi has been appreciated, and his house has become one great school of spirituality."

Monsignor Ersilio Tonini, the Archbishop of Macerata and Ravenna, wrote of Luigi: "I have known him very well, and I have been immediately spellbound by him. Two aspects particularly struck me, Luigi's serenity and his desire not to be pitied. Luigi had a great gift, a liberty of spirit—a liberty of mind. I have never seen anyone as happy as he. But there is another characteristic, the need to share his happiness, to encourage in others a deep relationship with God, for them to find happiness in pain . . . I can say that Luigi was one of the most beautiful souls I have ever met in my life . . ."

Luigi died at the age of 47 in Tolentino on March 26, 1979 and has become known by countless people throughout the world through the many books and materials written about him. The Bishop of Tolentino initiated the cause for his beatification on October 17, 1992.

59. Saint Lydwine of Schiedam
(1380-1433)

*L*YDWINE was born in the Netherlands, near the Hague, and was the only girl in a family of nine children. At Baptism she was given her name, which means "to suffer" in the Flemish language and "great patience" in the German tongue. The name was to be prophetic, since she was to suffer long and intensely in union with the Passion of our Saviour.

When she was old enough, Lydwine assisted her mother with the housework and became a clever worker. At the age of 15 there seems to have been nothing to distinguish Lydwine from other lively, healthy, and pretty girls of her age. She loved to ice skate, and when persuaded by her friends to join them in skating on a frozen canal, she went with them. She and her companions were just beginning to skate when a latecomer hurried to catch up and fell against Lydwine, causing her to fall against a piece of ice with such force that one of the ribs on her right side was broken.

People of the town offered advice on how to heal the fracture and reduce the pain, but when their remedies failed, renowned physicians were called in. These doctors prescribed medicines that only worsened her condition. A hard abscess developed, and as the physicians and others could not cure the girl's problem, they gradually abandoned her.

The pain became intolerable, so that Lydwine could find no relief either lying, sitting or standing. One day, when she could

141

bear the pain no longer, she threw herself from her couch and fell upon the knees of her father, who had been weeping as he sat nearby. This movement broke the abscess, but instead of releasing the infection externally, the abscess opened internally, forcing the infected matter to pour from Lydwine's mouth. The amount of the matter was so great that vessels used to catch the outpourings filled quickly. When they were emptied, they were quickly filled once again.

Unable to stand, Lydwine was forced to drag herself around on her knees—a practice that she continued for three years, until she was confined to bed for the rest of her life.

The wound under the rib gradually swelled and developed a gangrenous condition. All attempted remedies only caused the patient additional discomfort.

A tumor then appeared on Lydwine's shoulder; this too putrefied, causing almost unbearable neuritis. The disease also affected Lydwine's right arm, consuming the flesh to the bone. That arm became useless and prevented her from turning on her side. Violent neuralgic pains then began, together with a pounding noise in her head.

The girl's beauty that had attracted many potential suitors had now become pitifully lost. Lydwine's forehead became cleft from the hairline to the center of her nose. Her chin dropped under the lower lip, and her mouth became swollen. She lost the sight of her right eye, while the other became sensitive to light. For weeks she suffered from a violent toothache, then a severe inflammation of the throat nearly suffocated her and caused bleeding from the nose, mouth and ears. Lydwine's lungs and liver began to decay, and a cancer devoured her flesh.

Everyone who knew her soon realized that Lydwine's condition was supported by God, who had apparently chosen her as a victim soul. With the help of her confessor, she came to understand that her sufferings were not only intended to expiate the sins of others, living and dead, but would also draw down great benefits for the Church. She accepted her trials so willingly and patiently that she even said that if a single Hail Mary could gain her recovery, she would not utter it.

The sufferings of this young woman were intense and alarming, especially when her stomach ruptured and had to be held in place with wrappings. A cushion had to be placed above her stomach and pressed down to hold her internal organs in place. It was said that each time her position was changed, her body had to be bound with cloths—otherwise her body would literally have fallen to pieces.

Lydwine began to experience supernatural favors, including living without food or sleep. This became a source of interest to others, so that many people visited her and asked countless questions, all of which added to her trials.

During her final years, Lydwine was subject to epilepsy, apoplexy and a violent toothache. An ulcer developed in her breast, and she suffered nerve contractions that contorted her limbs.

From the first day of her injury on the ice until the day of her death, Lydwine's sufferings lasted for 38 years. She died on Easter Tuesday in the year 1433. Immediately the wounds of her body healed, the cleft in her forehead disappeared, and a heavenly sweetness was detected by many who came to pay their last respects.

Pope Benedict XIV wrote of St. Lydwine, "It seemed as if a whole army of diseases had invaded her body." St. Alphonsus Liguori wrote of her, "I know not whether there is to be met with among the annals of the Saints an instance of any other soul suffering so great affliction and desolation as did this holy virgin."

60. Venerable Maggiorino Vigolungo
(1904-1918)

LESSED James Alberione is the founder of the religious Order, the Paulines, which is also known as the Society of St. Paul. Early in his ministry he founded a small publishing house for the publishing and dispersing of religious materials. To help in this endeavor, he organized a group of boys in a vocational technical school. Among these was the exceptional Maggiorino, a boy who had been born on May 6, 1903 in Benevello, Italy to humble farm workers. He was a good-looking boy of lively intelligence who worked hard at being the first in his schoolwork and his games.

When Maggiorino was 12 years old, he met Fr. Alberione and was inspired to help in the publication of religious materials. He assisted the other boys with operating the machinery and joined them for prayer and schoolwork. When not engaged with working in "The Little Print Shop," he went onto the streets, handing out leaflets containing spiritual messages.

To Fr. Alberione, who was his spiritual director, Maggiorino once confided his constant dream: to become an apostle of the Catholic press, to become a priest, and then to become a saint. The boy once wrote, "With the grace of the Lord and the help of the Blessed Mother, I want to become a saint, a great saint, and a saint very soon." He was delighted with his vocation and grew each day in the love of God, being especially attracted to the Holy Eucharist. So determined was he to advance in virtue that he accepted as his motto, "Progress, a little every day."

After his 14th birthday, Maggiorino became seriously ill. Father Alberione asked him if he wanted to get well or go to Heaven, and the boy answered simply, "I desire to do the Will of God."

When it seemed that Maggiorino was not getting well, his parents brought him home. It was sometime later that he was diagnosed with pleurisy and then with meningitis. His friends became so worried about his condition that they joined in three days of intense prayer. However, it was apparently not God's Will that Maggiorino recover.

Maggiorino died on July 27, 1918 at the age of 14. His last words to his companions were, "Pray that we may find each other all together in Paradise."

Maggiorino's remains are kept in a vault in the Church of St. Paul in Alba. Pope John Paul II approved the Decree *Super Virtutibus* in 1988, elevating the young boy to the rank of Venerable.

61. Blessed Manuel Lozano Garrido
(1920-1971)

ANUEL was a healthy baby when he was born in Linares, Jaen, in the region of Andalusia, Spain. He was a normal youngster, and his religious education began at the age of nine. When he was a little older, he became active in an organization of charitable works known as Catholic Action, and, as he revealed, "I began almost as a boy to write in commercial papers."

During the Spanish Civil War of 1936-1939, when Manuel was 16 years old, he was entrusted with the solemn task of distributing the Holy Eucharist to various groups of Catholics who were in hiding because of the religious persecution that existed in Spain.

When it came time to select a career, it seemed natural for him to choose that of journalism. He wrote for the religious media, including the newspaper YA and the Associated Press. He was successful and productive, but then, at the age of 22, Manuel contracted spondylitis, a condition that inflames the vertebrae. From then on he endured pain and a rapidly increasing deformity of his back, which eventually necessitated his use of a wheelchair. In spite of the pain, Manuel continued to write articles for magazines and newspapers that centered on evangelization.

When Manuel slowly began to lose his sight, he did not let this or his painful deformity hinder his work—nor did he allow these disabilities to interfere with his zeal to use the media for the good of souls and of the Church. Despite his blindness, he continued to write intense articles and to dictate nine books to his sister, Lucy, and to friends. He was also a poet, the editor of hundreds of articles, the writer of stories and the founder of *Sinai,* a magazine for the sick. In recognition of his journalistic accomplishments, the Spanish Bishops' Conference in 1969 awarded him their most prestigious honor, the Bravo Award. In addition, he received 20 other literary and journalistic prizes.

Manuel used a wheelchair for 28 years and suffered for the last 10 years of his life. He died on November 3, 1971 at the age of 51. An investigation for the cause of his beatification began soon after. According to the postulator of his cause, all the documentation and testimonies that have been collected prove that Manuel Lozano Garrido led a virtuous and exemplary life. Already the cause has been graced with the first miracle of healing, that of a two-year-old Spanish boy who is today an international tennis umpire. Five doctors have confirmed the healing as being inexplicable.

The same publishing house that issued Manuel's books also published his biography, *Joy in Suffering,* which was written by the postulator of his cause, Reverend Rafael Higueras.

Manuel was beatified by Pope Benedict XVI on June 12, 2010.

62. BLESSED MARCEL CALLO (1921-1945)

ARCEL was born on the feast of the Immaculate Conception, December 8, 1921 at Rennes, France, one of nine children. As one of the older children, he was expected to help in the care and management of the household. He willingly helped his mother wash the dishes, straighten the house and wash and dress his younger brothers and sisters. He did all this with care and in good spirits.

After completing his primary studies at the age of 13, Marcel was apprenticed to a printer and willingly surrendered his salary to his mother to help with the needs of the family.

During his apprenticeship, Marcel disliked the improper stories told by his fellow workers, and he joined a Catholic organization where he found friends more to his liking. He was known among them for his ready laugh, his friendship and his religious interests.

When Marcel was 20 years old, he met and fell in love with a young lady. He was to say at that time, "One must master his heart before he can give it to the one that is chosen for him by Christ." He delayed kissing her for some time since, as his fiancée later wrote, "He had wanted to delay this gesture in order to thank God that we knew each other."

Marcel's life was interrupted on March 8, 1943 when World War II reached the city of Rennes with an aerial bombardment. Soon after, he was ordered to report to the Service of Obligatory Work in Germany where young Frenchmen were forced to work. Before leaving, Marcel told an aunt, "I will do everything possible to do well, because you know that it is not as a worker that I leave, but as a missionary."

While at Zella-Mehlis, Germany, Marcel reported to a factory that made artillery, which he learned would be used against the French people. Marcel suffered from homesickness, and for three months he fought a terrible depression. Although the workers were given some freedom, Marcel found it impossible to find a church that still offered Holy Mass, but he was able to find a room where Mass was secretly offered on Sundays. He was to write home: "Jesus made me to understand that the depression was not good. I had to keep busy with my friends, and then joy and relief would come back to me."

He began at once to organize a team of his Christian workers to pray, play cards, and take part in sports and other activities. He wrote home: "I believe I am still in Rennes in full activity. I give much and I receive much in return. When I do good things for others, I am satisfied."

For his French comrades, Marcel was able to arrange for a solemn Mass to be celebrated in their language, which was gratefully and enthusiastically attended.

The German officials eventually became aware of Marcel's religious activities, prompting them to arrest him on April 19, 1944. When asked by a friend why Marcel was being arrested, the agent responded, "Monsieur is too much of a Catholic."

Marcel freely admitted carrying on his religious activities and was taken to the prison in Gotha, where he continued his life of prayer and his interest in the condition of his companions. He once told his fellow prisoners, "It is in prayer that we find our strength." It is known that Marcel received his last Holy Communion when a friend secretly brought a consecrated Host to him in prison.

Marcel was later moved to the prison at Mathausen, where he

suffered for five months from general weakness, fever, swellings, bronchitis, malnutrition and dysentery—yet he never complained. He "expired softly like a lamb." It was the feast of St. Joseph, March 19, 1945, exactly two years from the day he had left France for Germany.

Pope John Paul II beatified Marcel Callo on October 4, 1987.

63. Blessed Margaret of Castello
(Bl. Margaret of Metola) (d. 1320)

ARGARET'S parents had joyfully anticipated the birth of their first child, but the event turned into a veritable tragedy when the newborn was found to be blind, hunchbacked, dwarfed, and lame. Her right leg was much shorter than the left, which was also malformed, and she is described quite forthrightly by contemporary biographers as being "ugly."

The parents, being of position and wealth, were overwhelmed with disappointment, anger, and loathing and attempted to keep the infant and her deformities secret. Since they wanted nothing to do with the child, she was entrusted to a servant, who saw to Margaret's Baptism and the choice of a name.

Because Margaret, at an early age, was given to prayer and visits to the castle's chapel, the father decided to force her to be a recluse. He had a room built beside the church with a window opening into the church and another small window opening outside, through which food could be passed. After she was placed in this room, a mason bricked the doorway. Margaret was six years old at the time.

During the 13th year of her imprisonment, when the father's territory was threatened with invasion, the parents went to the safety of Mercatello, taking Margaret with them. But there Margaret was again imprisoned, this time in an underground vault. When news reached the parents that cures were taking place in the city of Castello at the tomb of the Franciscan tertiary, Fra

Giacomo, Margaret was taken there. But after many hours, when a cure was not effected, the parents did the unbelievable and abandoned their daughter there. One can only imagine the grief this caused Margaret when she learned of their rejection of her. However, it is known that she never blamed her parents or spoke unkindly of them.

For a time, Margaret was looked after by villagers, until a community of nuns accepted her. After a few years, when the community's rule was relaxed, the nuns felt ashamed that Margaret continued to observe the rule strictly. To relieve their consciences, Margaret was asked to leave.

Not realizing the conditions in the convent, the villagers thought Margaret had been expelled for not adjusting herself to community life. As a result, she was ridiculed by villagers, including even children. It is said that even in church she was the object of sneering words. But when the situation at the convent became known, Margaret's reputation rose to a high level.

Realizing that Margaret always had a desire to join a religious Order, the Third Order of St. Dominic accepted her, and she became a devoted member, observing the Rule, practicing various penances and fasts, and ministering to anyone in need. One contemporary biographer relates: "No sick person was too far away for her to limp to, no hour of the day or night was ever too inconvenient for her to hasten to those in agony."

Margaret was accepted into various homes, and she once heard someone describe the frightful conditions at the local prison. From then on she persuaded her fellow tertiaries to help her in ministering to the unfortunates there. In addition to bringing clothing, food and medicine to the prisoners, Margaret was successful in bringing many prisoners back to the good graces of the Church. When one inmate was particularly obstinate, Margaret began praying, and as she prayed, she slowly levitated. When she descended to the ground, the prisoner begged for her prayers.

It is said that, although blind, Margaret could see visions of Our Lord. During her lifetime she was known to have effected numerous and marvelous miracles and to have counseled many in the ways of prayer and the acceptance of hardships.

After receiving the Sacraments and other comforts of the Church, and with friars and her fellow tertiaries beside her bed, Margaret died at the beginning of the year 1320. She was 33 years old. She was entombed in one of the chapels of the Dominican Church, but before her interment there, a crippled child was cured. Unable to walk or talk previously, the child now declared that she had been cured through Margaret's prayers. After the funeral, more than 200 affidavits were received testifying to permanent cures received through Margaret's intercession.

Margaret was beatified by Pope Paul V in 1609. Dressed in the black and white habit of the Dominican order, Margaret's incorrupt body is now seen in a glass sarcophagus in the chapel of the School for the Blind in Citta di Castello, Italy.

64. VENERABLE MARI CARMEN GONZALEZ-VALERIO (1930-1939)

DESCRIPTIONS of this nine-year-old reveal that she was profoundly sincere, with a clear and alert intelligence—that she had a sound judgment, persevering fervor, exquisite sensibility and always took responsibility for her actions. Yet she was a completely normal girl with a strong character who enjoyed playing with dolls and eating sweets.

Mari Carmen was born April 16, 1930 in Madrid to a family of deep spirituality. The happiness of her birth was soon marred when the infant became seriously ill. For this reason she was baptized immediately in her home. According to the custom of the time, she received the Sacrament of Confirmation when she was only two years old and received her First Holy Communion when she was six. Her mother noticed that after receiving her First Holy Communion "she began to show signs of real sanctity." From then on she began to attend Mass and receive Holy Communion almost every day.

Six years after her birth the Spanish Civil War began, with its religious persecution against Catholics and the Church. The father was arrested and killed, but Mari Carmen's mother and her five children were able to seek asylum in the Belgian Embassy. At this time, Mari Carmen tried to console her mother by suggesting, "Don't be upset. Let's say the Rosary and recall Jesus' wounds."

This very spiritual child had forgiven her father's assassins, and she faithfully prayed for the conversion of Azaña, the Pres-

ident of the Republic—who, she reasoned, was the symbol of
the whole religious persecution. Mari Carmen prayed the
Rosary of the Divine Wounds every day for his conversion,
which occurred sometime later.

The spirituality of Mari Carmen is noted in her "diary,"
which she kept in an envelope sealed with adhesive tape. On the
envelope she wrote three times, "Private." After her death,
among the little notations was found: "*Viva España. Viva Cristo
Rey*," words that were on the lips of many martyrs during the
Spanish civil war. Also found was this notation: "I surrendered
myself in the parish church of the Buen Pastor, April 6, 1939."
Her surrender was accepted, since the infection that claimed her
life began 15 days later.

While at school in Zalla, Mari Carmen contracted scarlet fever,
accompanied by an infection of the ear and the mastoid. The
infection, unfortunately, degenerated into septicemia that settled
in the heart and kidneys. A mastoid operation and a thrombec-
tomy were performed, but when Mari Carmen did not improve
after surgery, the doctors knew her condition was hopeless.

She once told her mother that "To be a saint you have to
mortify yourself." This the child did most admirably. And then,
when the mother said she would ask the Child Jesus for a cure,
Mari Carmen interrupted, "No, Mama, I don't ask for that. I
ask that His Will be done."

One of her nurses tells us, "When they brought her from the
clinic she was suffering a great deal with septicemia . . . she had
open sores. We had to give her blood transfusions twice a day
and many injections. Some days there were more than 20. She
also suffered from colitis, which she had very severely . . . " In
addition to suffering from her illnesses, which she accepted
peacefully and willingly, Mari Carmen was often given only
bland food to eat, which it was thought would cure the colitis.

When asked what she would like to eat, she replied, "Whatever you think best." Often, before a painful treatment, she would ask everyone present to pray the Creed and the Our Father. Then she would submit without a word.

Mari Carmen suffered other complications, especially phlebitis, which produced gangrenous wounds on her thighs. Simply moving the bed sheets caused her torments. She was also feverish and suffered from insomnia. Sometimes she could not help but cry out in pain, but afterwards she would always say, "You, doctor, and everybody, please excuse me."

Doctor Antonio Martin Cadenin tells of her heroic patience: "During all that time and despite her nine years, this little girl endured all that pain and suffering with a truly exemplary resignation. It was extraordinary to observe how, when we would try some remedy or apply an injection, very painful procedures, especially in her state, all we had to do was to say 'Jesus' in order for her to endure it without complaint and without moving, something we doctors had never encountered in one so young."

Mari Carmen often predicted that the Blessed Mother would come for her on the feast day of Our Lady of Mount Carmel, July 16, but when July 17 dawned, she sat up in her bed—something she had been unable to do—and announced joyfully, "Today I am going to die. Today I am going to Heaven!" And she was delighted that she would soon be reunited with her father.

Moments before dying, Mari Carmen looked at her relatives gathered around her bed and advised them, "Love one another." She then asked if they heard the beautiful singing. Her grandmother told her the singers were Angels, to which the child answered, "Yes, indeed. They are the Angels who have come for me." She then announced with a smile, "I am going to Heaven. I am going without passing through Purgatory because I have been a martyr at the hands of the doctors. I die a martyr." She then said, "Jesus, Mary, and Joseph, grant that when I die, I die in peace and my soul comes to be with you." She died soon after. She was nine years old.

After Mari Carmen's death, her face, which had been badly disfigured by her illness, immediately changed so that everyone said she had regained her former beauty. Everyone was enraptured by the change and by the sweet aroma that filled the room, although there was not a flower present.

Little Mari Carmen was buried in the church of the monastery of the Discalced Carmelites in Aravaca, Madrid. The diocesan process for her beatification was opened 22 years later. In 1996 she was declared Venerable.

65. Servant of God Maria a Columna Cimadevilla y Lopez-Doriga
(1952-1962)

THIS impressive name was given the child when she was born on February 17, 1952 in Madrid, Spain, but she was always lovingly called Puma. As a child she was affectionate, reflective, nostalgic and sensitive by nature but soon developed a deep love of Church and neighbor. She was a normal little girl in all respects, who loved to play games. She was different in that she always ended the games before her opponent lost. In this way she saved her opponent from the disappointment at not having won. The child practiced charity in this and many other ways. She was exceptional in that she also practiced little acts of mortification and accepted everything as coming from the hands of God, especially when she was four years old and began to suffer various childhood ailments.

When asked what she wanted to be when she grew up, Puma's answer was amazing: she replied that she wanted to be the little companion of the Child Jesus. The Sisters at school taught her well. When her dress, veil and flowered crown were being prepared for her First Holy Communion, she surprised everyone by saying in all seriousness that clothes were of no importance, only union with Jesus mattered. She received the Holy Sacrament for the first time on May 15, 1959 with deep reverence. From then on, Puma wanted to receive Our Lord as often as possible.

About this time, Puma's physical condition began to deteriorate. The parents suspected a mere childhood illness, but examinations and tests revealed that the six-year-old was suffering from Hodgkin's disease, a painful and malignant disorder of the lymph nodes which often involves other organs. It produces fatigue, loss of weight, fever and pain.

Puma suspected the serious nature of her illness, but her reaction surprised her parents; she whispered, "I offer my life to Jesus." Her willing and pleasant acceptance of her forthcoming death inspired the doctors, nurses, and her many visitors who came seeking encouragement in their own trials.

Puma was particularly fond of the lives of the Saints, and she contemplated their graces and sufferings. She once mentioned to her mother that, like the Saints, she must suffer for her little transgressions, but that it was good that Jesus gave her sufferings since God the Father had sent sufferings to His own Son. "All should be joyfully accepted."

On days when Puma could not receive the Holy Eucharist because of her physical sufferings, she nevertheless prayed the Rosary with her mother, even though her little body was exhausted from fever and pain. Her sufferings were truly heroic. Fully realizing that she would soon die, she remained calm, sweet, smiling and completely resigned to the Will of God.

As if her sufferings were not enough, she practiced voluntary sacrifices, such as delaying a refreshment offered during a feverish night, accepting it only in the morning.

When Puma heard of an organization known as the Union of Infirm Missionaries, which consisted of sick persons who offered their sufferings for foreign missionaries, she joined it, being content that her sufferings were being joined to those of Jesus on the Cross. Her prayer was that the Heavenly Father would increase vocations to missionary fields.

When Puma's illness had progressed to its final stage, one of her doctors testified, "I have followed with great care the physical condition of this nine-year-old child . . . Everyone loved to enter her room because of her angelic smile. She never spoke of her illness, neither of the pain, neither of death, but rather, of her longing for Heaven, all of which indicated the greatness of her soul. Were it not for the results of laboratory tests, one would not believe she endured fever or pain. She impressed me profoundly."

Puma died on March 6, 1962 at the age of ten and was buried in the cemetery of Carabanchel. Her classmates sang during the funeral Mass, while the Sisters of the hospital carried the casket to its crypt. When the Process of Beatification was initiated, the relics were transferred to the parish church of St. Ginés, where Puma had received her First Holy Communion and where she had so often received the Sacraments.

The application for the beatification of Maria a Columna Cimadevilla y Lopez-Doriga was accepted by the Congregation for the Causes of Saints in 1986.

66. Blessed Maria Bartolomea Bagnesi
(1514-1577)

MARIA Bagnesi was born into a wealthy Florentine family who found it necessary to place the infant in the care of a foster mother. Unfortunately, the infant received inadequate care and poor nutrition, which proved so detrimental that Maria was never able in later life to eat a normal meal.

Maria would have followed her elder sister into the religious life except for the death of the mother. Maria, who was then not quite 18 years old, was obliged to assume the supervision of the father's household, although always hoping to enter a Carmelite convent. Unknown to Maria, her father arranged a marriage for her, which so shocked and grieved her that she suffered a complete breakdown of her health.

She became a bedridden invalid with problems that included pleurisy, asthma, kidney disease, and conditions affecting her eyes, ears, head, stomach and intestines. She also experienced temporary blindness and deafness. Her sufferings were increased when she was subjected to revolting and painful remedies prescribed by her physicians and by charlatans employed by her father. It is said that her condition became so critical that on eight occasions she received the Last Sacraments.

The father finally abandoned hope for her health and marriage when Maria was 32 years old. He then recommended that she join the Third Order of St. Dominic. For a short time she returned to relatively good health, but then her previous afflictions returned with such intensity that she was obliged to return to her bed.

Although she suffered intensely, Maria was never heard to complain, and she continued to exercise a wonderful influence on a great many people. Her sanctity was such that she was enabled to read the hearts of her visitors and was granted a share in heavenly knowledge and an advanced spirit of prayer.

In addition to her sufferings from illness, it became later known that a tyrannical servant who cared for the invalid had afflicted Maria with various forms of abuse, which Maria had patiently endured for 24 years.

Maria died at the age of 63, after suffering as an invalid for 45 years. The Carmelites, who had been unable to accept Maria Bagnesi as a member because of her poor health, provided a tomb for her in the chapel of their convent. Years later, when her body was transferred to the cloister, it was found to be incorrupt.

Many miracles were performed through the intercession of Maria Bagnesi, especially one in favor of the future St. Mary Magdalene de' Pazzi (d. 1607), who would spend three and a half months in the convent infirmary. When St. Mary Magdalene asked to be taken to the shrine of Maria Bagnesi, she was immediately cured. Later she beheld Maria in the glorious company of Our Lord and His holy Mother.

Maria Bagnesi was solemnly beatified by Pope Pius VII in 1804.

67. Venerable Maria Carmelina Leone
(1923-1940)

ARIA'S parents were known throughout the neighborhood for their intense piety, from which Maria benefited, displaying since early childhood a constant and faithful love of prayer. During her early childhood, the parents realized that Maria was specially called to a higher level of virtue and entrusted her to the protection of Our Lady of Mount Carmel. From then on the child was faithful in wearing the brown scapular, which was for her the beloved garment of the Virgin Mary.

Under the direction of her spiritual advisor, Maria advanced quickly in the way of perfection, and she became active in teaching the Faith among the people of her district, as well as serving as a catechist in the church of the Jesuits.

Maria was adept at embroidery, and after studying at a trade school, she worked as a tailor. She would have liked to enter the religious life, but this dream had to be set aside when it was discovered that she had tuberculosis. For a time she was treated in a sanatorium, but when she did not respond to medication, she was returned home to die. Maria is said to have lived in a continual dialogue with God and the Blessed Virgin, and she was a contemplative according to the Carmelite spirit.

Toward the end of her life she began to predict future events, including the day of her own death, and she once advised her family and friends, "When I am up there in Heaven, call me in all your needs. I will be present, and I will pray for all of you."

Maria suffered heroically until she succumbed to the disease on October 10, 1940, being called thereafter the "holy, afflicted one." After her burial, a spontaneous popular cult developed, with countless people visiting her grave and the home of her parents. Many were spiritually enriched by these visits and edified by the life of this simple but saintly 17-year-old girl. Maria soon became known throughout Sicily and beyond, with the devotion of her clients being rewarded with favors of all sorts.

The introduction of the cause for her beatification was soon opened, with the Decree of Heroic Virtue being made on April 8, 1997, which awarded Maria Carmelina the title of Venerable. The "holy, afflicted one" now awaits beatification.

68. SERVANT OF GOD
MARIA CAROLINA SCAMPONE (1877-1951)

AROLINA'S life was a very sad and complicated one. She was the wife of a difficult husband, then a widow, an indigent woman, and even a prisoner during World War II. She was also a Carmelite tertiary, the mother of five and, in the end, a resident in a Roman hospice for the aged poor. A simple, devout woman, Carolina lived in a spirit of confidence in God, recognizing the cross as the source of grace and spiritual growth.

Carolina came from a devout family, being born in a town situated between Rome and Naples. Later the family relocated to a small town named Selvacava. Her family participated in the devotions related to the liturgical year and observed days of fasting and penance. The holy days were observed with special celebrations.

According to the custom of the time, Carolina's father selected a young man for her to marry. At first she resisted, but then, in obedience, she consented to the marriage. Her husband was not a devout man, but in the beginning he participated in the family Rosary. In time he became nervous and irritable, with a fierce temper. Carolina suffered greatly from his abuse but remained patient and long-suffering. When he became ill with cancer, Carolina tended him with great care. After his death, she was left with five children to support. For the first time in her life she went looking for work. During the winter she joined the olive pickers, and in the summer she went into the hills, gathering wood, which she sold each evening.

One of her neighbors recalled: "She was poor, but she gave whatever she had to those who knocked at her door, depriving herself in the process . . . She was counselor and teacher to the people of our town. Yet, frequently, I saw her in tears, recommending herself to Providence, because she did not have enough bread to provide for her ailing father and her children."

Carolina's only daughter, Erminia, announced one day that she had a religious vocation and entered the Sisters of the Poor of St. Catherine of Siena. One son died after an illness, two emigrated to Argentina, and her son Felice joined the Italian national police force. For a time he was able to help his mother financially, but unfortunately, Felice died in an accident, which caused Carolina to suffer an epileptic seizure, a disorder that was to plague her the rest of her life.

With all her children gone, she again resorted to menial jobs, when another affliction visited her in the form of an eye condition. She was treated by a doctor as long as she could pay for his services. She then resigned herself to losing the sight in the eye.

More troubles visited Carolina when World War II erupted. When the Germans retreated, they took some of the villagers with them, including Carolina. The villagers lived in the caves of Monte Casino, where aerial bombardment deafened them. A companion at the time reported that "Carolina was our comfort. Still impressed on my mind is her image: comforting us, advising us not to lose courage because the Lord would help and support us with His grace . . . I could not understand how she could be so calm because we were overcome with fright."

Carolina was eventually imprisoned and sent to a concentration camp. She was terribly hungry and sick during the final months of the War, suffering not only from her epileptic attacks, but also from a rash that caused a high fever and great discomfort. After she was set free, she endured two painful operations and remained two years in the ward for the chronically ill, where she endured various inconveniences and where even meals were often forgotten. Carolina never complained but regarded these difficulties as opportunities for spiritual growth.

Transferred to the Institute Santa Maria della Providenza in Rome, she lived there six years. Her nurse, Sister Maria Barca, remembered: "In 1944 I had the honor of welcoming Maria Carolina Scampone into our house. She was very good; she spoke little, but her face was absorbed in prayer. During her long suffering, there was never a word of complaint. She was the best in the ward. I recognized her as a soul of outstanding virtue."

Carolina became a Carmelite Third Order member on her deathbed and died after a five-day agony. She was buried in Rome's Campo Verano cemetery. She has since become widely known, with favors of all sorts being reported as a result of her intercession.

69. SERVANT OF GOD
MARIA CRISTINA OGIER (1955-1974)

MARIA Ogier was especially devoted to the well-being of others, especially the missions, the unborn and the sick. What this young girl of only 19 years started as an act of charity is still continuing today by those who admired her ideals and the sufferings which she offered up for the welfare of the Church.

She was born in Florence, Italy, the only child of Dr. Henry Ogier, an obstetrician and gynecologist, and Gina Matteoni, both devout Catholics. Maria was a healthy child until the age of four, when she contracted an illness common to children. But unlike the others, she did not recover completely. Eventually she began to drag her right foot, which resulted in numerous examinations. The diagnosis was a devastating one: a tumor on the brain. Because of her tender years it was thought best not to operate, since her survival was uncertain. Instead, she was prepared for her First Holy Communion, which she received on April 30, 1961.

Four months later, accompanied by her spiritual director, Don Setti, and her parents, Maria went to Lourdes for the first time. She was taken in a wheelchair and frequently drank the miraculous water. Later, on several occasions she was privileged to visit Padre Pio.

Maria was well for a time, but at the age of seven she once again began to limp slightly. Still, she never underwent the delicate operation that might have cured the condition. When asked how she felt, she replied, "There are many people suffering more than I am, and they are poor and I am short of nothing." When her mother noticed that she did not pray for herself, she asked Maria if she wanted to pray to the Madonna for a cure. Maria replied, "No, Mamma, I pray for the salvation of the world."

She attended school when she was able, and at the age of 13 she helped organize prayer groups at two churches. Under the direction of her spiritual advisor, she advanced quickly in virtue and in the desire to practice charity. At the age of 14 or 15, she joined Don Setti's group, which visited hospitals, prisons and the House of Hope for needy families. The visits to the hospitals inspired Maria in the choice of her life's work. She decided to become a doctor so she could help the sick.

Although this dream was never realized, Maria was to accomplish much in this field, and in an extraordinary manner. A doctor-priest of the Capuchin Order was visiting Florence for a refresher course in obstetrics under the direction of her father, Dr. Ogier. The priest was explaining the difficulty in the mission field of the Amazon in getting patients to the missionaries' hospital. The sick and wounded were transported several miles by canoes, but many of the sick died on the way. He announced, "What is needed is a boat with all the facilities for casualties and first aid."

Maria's charity was immediately aroused. It was said that she never saw a person in need whom she did not help by her charity. This was a new field of endeavor, and she immediately began to write letters to everyone she knew—to various religious organizations, to newspapers, churches, businesses and schools. Her persistence was rewarded. Even though suffering frequent headaches and difficulty in walking, she had plans for the boat drawn up, and in time the costs were met. Then, with the help of her father and his friends, the boat was fitted with all the latest testing equipment and medical supplies. On the day it was given to the Capuchin Order, a picture was taken of the family in front of the boat, which was named the *Maria Cristina* in her honor. It continues to sail the Amazon River at the publication of this book. The building and outfitting of this boat proves that it is truly amazing what one person can do, even though suffering from a malignant condition.

Maria received Holy Communion every day. Each night after the family Rosary, her mother would find her on her knees. To a suggestion that she go to bed, Maria once replied, "I must still pray for the whole world, for the missions, for Don Setti, for the sick . . ."

She had a great love of Our Lady and was attracted to St. Francis. After reading his life she applied to and was admitted into the Franciscan Third Order. Still dreaming of a medical career, Maria enrolled in the Faculty of Medicine at the University and attended several lectures, but she was becoming unusually tired and weak, absent-minded and inattentive. The tumor in her brain remained the same size, and her leg still dragged, but another difficulty was added when it became necessary for Maria to support her right hand with her left. One day after attending Mass and receiving Holy Communion, as was her custom, Maria suffered a bulbar paralysis, which ended her life.

During her 19 years Maria had wanted to establish houses for the sick, where there would be better living conditions and which would be maintained by personnel who had good attitudes toward the sick. After her death, a foundation was established by those who were inspired by her ideals. The nursing homes she envisioned were established, as well as a day hospital and the means to re-fuel the boat, the *Maria Cristina*. In her memory a home for young girls was founded, as well as homes for pregnant women who suffered from serious economic and social difficulties. In 1986 the Center was visited by Pope John Paul II, who spoke with Dr. Ogier about his saintly daughter.

70. SAINT MARIA MAZZARELLO (1837-1881)

ARIA Mazzarello was born the eldest of ten children in Mornese, Italy, where her father had a small farm. At an early age, she was obliged to help in the fields, and it is said that as she grew older she could outwork any of the male field hands and that her yield was always the largest. She is known to have attended daily Mass despite even inclement weather, and then to have reported promptly to the fields.

When she was 15 years old, a typhus epidemic invaded Mornese. Since Maria was strong and hard working, she helped many of the afflicted to regain their health, but then she herself contracted the disease. At times she was almost at the point of death. She recovered, but she retained a certain weakness, which prevented her from returning to the fields.

Looking about for another means of helping her family, Maria with her sister and a friend, Petronilla, began to study sewing from the best tailor in the town. Afterward, they opened a little place where they taught little girls to sew and to make little things for sale. Although Maria had had little formal education, she learned the catechism and began giving lessons to the children, as well as encouraging them to attend Mass and receive the Sacraments. In addition Maria sponsored little sporting events, excursions and prayers, all of which attracted more young girls to her classes.

While Maria was busy training and teaching girls, St. John Bosco was having the same success among boys in Turin.

While traveling on a train, Don Bosco learned from one of the passengers about the work accomplished by Maria Mazzarello. He visited her on October 7, 1864—which was a momentous event for the town, since Don Bosco was already well known for his holiness. Maria was full of admiration when she heard his sermons, and she profited much from his instructions.

When Don Bosco noticed that many of the older girls were excellent candidates for the religious life, he founded—together with Maria—the Daughters of Mary Auxiliatrix, also known as the female branch of the Salesians. The community was approved by Pope Pius IX in 1857. The Salesian Order is regarded as the second largest religious community in the world and is present in 75 countries.

Maria was elected Mother General and served for ten years, until she contracted pleurisy, an inflammation of the membranes surrounding the lungs. Maria died of this condition on May 14, 1881 and was canonized by Pope Pius XII in 1938.

71. Venerable Matthew Talbot
(1856-1925)

ATTHEW Talbot was born in the small seaside village of Clontarf, which is located two miles from Dublin, Ireland. He was the second of twelve children. During an age when compulsory school attendance was rarely enforced, Matthew was enrolled at the Christian Brothers School, where he attended for only one year. During this time he was taught to read and write, and he learned his prayers and the truths of the Faith in preparation for his reception of the Sacraments. After this, he began working in Dublin as a messenger boy for a wine merchant. Though not yet a teenager, he soon began to sample his employer's product. His sister, Mrs. Mary Andrews, tells that "He learned to take alcoholic drink to excess." His father learned about this and found Matthew a position as a messenger boy in the Port and Docks Board Office, where the father also worked.

Another of Matthew's sisters reports, "He told me himself that he sold his boots and shirt to get drink, and he used to get drink on credit, often having his wages spent in advance . . . I heard him say (after his conversion) that even when drinking he was devout in his mind to the Blessed Virgin and used to say an odd Hail Mary, and he attributed his conversion to this."

In spite of his heavy drinking, Matthew was a good and steady workman. While employed as a hodman for a bricklayer, he accomplished more in half an hour than other workers managed in an hour. In time, he became known as the "best hodman in Dublin," but there were days when he failed to report for work, being totally intoxicated.

Since his income was insufficient to maintain his excessive drinking habit, Matthew sometimes supplemented his wages by collecting and selling empty bottles and by collecting tips for holding horses outside Carolan's Pub. Matthew was an alcoholic who carelessly lost his self-respect, refused to listen to the appeals of his mother, and drank not only his earnings, but also any money he and his companions could come by honestly or otherwise.

One day he was without money and was waiting at the corner of William Street and North Strand for his friends, who were leaving work with their wages. He expected to be invited by them to have a drink, but when they all passed him by without the expected offer, Matthew had a great deal to think about and returned home. After serious reflection, he told his mother that he was going to "take the pledge."

Matthew made his Confession at Clonliffe College and took the pledge not to drink for three months. The following morning, Matthew received the Holy Eucharist for the first time in years. He became a changed man, working regularly, avoiding his former companions and spending more time in church. The inclination to return to his former habits stayed with him, and he struggled to keep the pledge. When the three months expired, he renewed the pledge for life.

Still working as a hodman, Matthew spent every free moment in prayer. He was never heard to swear, and he observed fasts and slept on a broad plank with a solid lump of wood for a pillow. He attended Mass daily and joined the Franciscan Third Order. Since he no longer squandered his income on alcohol, he gave freely to his mother, the poor, and to religious organizations, especially the missions.

Matthew read a great many books that were recommended to him and developed a great devotion to St. Teresa of Avila and St. Thérèse of Lisieux. In one of these books he wrote these thoughtful words: "Three things I cannot escape: the eye of God, the voice of conscience, the stroke of death. In company, guard your tongue. In your family, guard your temper. When alone, guard your thoughts." Another time he wrote: "In prayer we speak to God; in spiritual reading and sermons God speaks to us."

Matthew is described as a man always in good humor and friendly with everyone, and he became a man of deep virtue, wearing neat but old clothes, living frugally and attending daily Mass. He was frequently seen praying the Rosary. So prayerful was he that youngsters in the neighborhood began referring to him as "Holy Joe."

One day Matthew gave away his pipe and tobacco and never smoked again. Added to his ever-present craving for alcohol, Matthew suffered the penance of additionally depriving himself of nicotine. He once confided to a friend that it cost him more to give up tobacco than to give up alcohol. In addition to this, he also observed numerous fasts, ate sparingly at other times, spent hours at night in prayer, and for many years wore a penitential chain around his waist.

During the last years of his life, Matthew suffered from kidney and heart ailments. He also suffered at times from great weakness of body. Then too, he developed a difficulty in breathing, no doubt caused by his years of heavy drinking and smoking. After one hospitalization, he was told by the doctors that his condition was so serious that he might die suddenly of his heart condition. That is exactly what took place on June 7, 1925 while Matthew Talbot was walking to Mass.

Six years after his death, the first inquiry into his life and virtues began. Another inquiry took place in 1948. During these inquiries, 68 people who had known Matthew Talbot gave depositions concerning his former alcoholic dependency, his courageous reform, and his virtuous and penitential life of 41 years.

Matthew Talbot was declared Venerable on October 3, 1975.

72. Servant of God Montserrat Grases
(1941-1959)

AMED for the shrine of Our Lady of Montserrat, a popular place of pilgrimage in Spain, this young girl was one of nine children and was known affectionately among family and friends as "Montse." Her mother once wrote: "We taught the children from the cradle to say some simple prayers, to develop a relationship with the Child Jesus, to have devotion to Our Lady, to accept and offer up pain, to struggle against one's own little defects, to help each other . . ." The mother concluded that "what happened in Montse's soul was because God wanted it. It was the result of her correspondence to grace. . . . She had no guile of any kind."

As she grew up, Montse had many and varied interests. She played ball and other sports, she received honors in piano and music theory, and she taught catechism to children. She loved tennis matches, mountain climbing, and even did a little acting. She loved to sing, swim, cycle, and dance the Sardanas, a traditional festive dance in which several people in a circle hold hands and dance to slow rhythmic music.

After a skiing trip, when she and her friends were running home, Montse had to stop because of an intense pain in her left leg. Since she continued to limp, a doctor was consulted; he prescribed vitamins. But when the pain persisted, she was told to wear a knee-guard. When the pain abated, Montse continued her normal activities and her usual prayers. These consisted of daily Mass, a half hour of mental prayer in the morning and another half hour in the evening, as well as all three parts of the Rosary.

After a second doctor was consulted, x-rays revealed a tumorous mass. Finally the diagnosis was confirmed. Montse had Ewing's Sarcoma, a malignant and irreversible cancer of the bone. The only treatment available at the time was radiation; this would prove to be a painful experience.

Montse told a companion, "I am ready to put up with whatever comes. . . . I am very afraid of suffering, and the doctors frighten me . . . but if God sends me more suffering, He will help me a lot." Another time, when she was seen kneeling before the image of Our Lady of Montserrat, she was heard to say, "Whatever you want."

During a visit with her friends, Montse seemed perfectly happy and was singing peacefully. She then remarked, "I really am at peace. I want God's will. This is the second time I gave myself to God. I have already done it once before." The pain, she said, was a "purification to get to Heaven." Montse was never heard to complain, and she seemed so serene that one would have doubted she was experiencing pain.

When a church group planned a trip to Rome, the members of the group insisted that Montse join them. She seemed well and happy during the pilgrimage and never complained, so that on her return home she was asked how she felt. To this Montse replied, "It is as if a mad dog were biting me all the time."

Later, it became increasingly difficult for fresh dressings to be applied to her badly swollen leg. After the inflammation burst and the bandages were removed, bits of flesh adhered to the dressings. The application of gauze and other bandages was a very painful procedure since there were large numbers of ulcers, and small hemorrhages occurred.

In spite of her pain, Montse resisted taking sedatives or anything that would alleviate the pain. She reasoned that the medication would make her sleep and would diminish her suffering, thereby interrupting the pain that she was offering to Our Lord for the Pope, her family and for others whom she mentioned.

Finally the time came when even the sheet touching Montse's leg was unbearable. To prevent this, a kind of cage was constructed so that the linen would not touch her. And every time the dressing was changed, a towel had to be placed beneath the leg to absorb the liquid that seeped from the wound.

Every day a priest would visit to bring Montse the Blessed Sacrament. She was extremely grateful for this and frequently exclaimed, "Without the Eucharist I could not live!"

Montse's father finally decided that it was time for her to receive the Sacrament of Anointing of the Sick. Afterward, Montse remarked, "I am really looking forward to going . . ." When her mother said that perhaps Our Lord wished her to continue helping souls, Montse replied, "Then I don't mind a few more days, or whenever Our Lord wills." During her last days she was heard to repeat: "Whenever You like, wherever You like, as You like . . ." Finally on Holy Thursday, March 26, 1959, as she clutched her crucifix, Montse went to her reward.

The Congregation for the Causes of Saints issued a decree on May 15, 1992 declaring the validity of the process for beatification. Montse's remains are kept at Bonaigua Residence Hall in Barcelona, where they are visited by many who admire her heroic life and her admirable degree of spirituality.

73. VENERABLE NICHOLAS HORNER
(d. 1590)

WHEN Elizabeth I was Queen of England (1558-1603), priests were considered traitors, and those who hid or aided them were liable to be severely punished. Living in London at the time was a tailor named Nicholas Horner, "a good and perfect Catholic, a man of plain and just dealing," who was apprehended for harboring priests.

For his crime of protecting priests, Nicholas was imprisoned in a detention place known as Newgate. Even though his leg had been seriously injured, the jailors clamped irons on both the prisoner's legs. The irons aggravated the condition to such an extent that amputation of the injured leg was inevitable.

Afraid that his pain during the amputation would give scandal to his fellow prisoners, Nicholas prayed fervently to Almighty God. While all was being prepared for surgery, a good priest who was in prison, called "Mr. Hewett," came forward and consoled the patient with a meditation about the sufferings of Christ during His passion. Then "holding the head of Nicholas betwixt his hands whilst it was adoing [the amputation]," the priest assisted him, and Nicholas endured the ordeal courageously. In the *Acts of English Martyrs*, it is recorded:

> But afterwards when it was cut off, it pleased God to give Nicholas such patience that he not only comforted the other Catholics that were there prisoners, but also drove the surgeons and other strangers that

beheld the same into admiration. For whilst it was in cutting off, he being made to sit on a form neither bound nor holden by any violence, neither offered to stir nor used any impatient screech or cries, but wringing his hands in very good order, often said, "Jesus, increase my patience."

Unfortunately, the wound of the amputation was slow in healing, so that Nicholas endured intense pain for almost 12 months. On learning of his condition, many outside petitioned for his release, which was granted—but Nicholas was again apprehended. When he refused to reveal the number and the names of priests who had found lodging in his home, he was hung by the wrists until he was almost dead.

During his next court appearance Nicholas was condemned when two witnesses testified that he had once sewn a jerkin for a priest. He was then condemned to death. Within a few days, Nicholas was hanged on a gibbet, having a title set above his head. As was the custom, he was taken down when he was almost dead, and his body, while he still lived, was drawn and quartered. Venerable Nicholas Horner suffered martyrdom at Smithfield on March 4, 1590.

74. Blessed Notker Balbulus (840-912)

ORN of noble Swiss parents in the city of Elgg, Switzerland, Blessed Notker, while still a small child, was sent to be educated in the Benedictine monastery school of St. Gall. It was hoped that his health would improve there and that somehow the monks would correct his stammering. While in his teens, Notker decided to stay at St. Gall's and become a monk. He impressed his colleagues and those who came to know of him so much that he was described as "weakly in body but not in mind, stammering of tongue but not of intellect, pressing forward boldly in things divine—a vessel filled with the Holy Ghost without equal in his time."

The holy monk served his community as librarian and then as guest master, and then began writing prose and poetry, so that he is regarded by many as the greatest poet of the Middle Ages. In addition, he studied music and became so accomplished that he became a noted teacher in the monastic school, despite his speech impediment.

Notker also composed music and is now considered to be the first musical composer of German stock. His fame is based on more than 38 Sequences which he composed. These are hymns based on rhythmical prose, originating in the ninth century, that are sung or read before the reading of the Gospel in the Traditional Latin Mass.

The latter years of Notker's life were spent in prayer and in preparation for death. He died of a fever in the midst of his brethren after giving them his blessing.

Notker was so beloved by the monks of his abbey that for a long time after his death they could not speak of him without shedding tears. The Holy See confirmed the cult of Blessed Notker in 1512 by permitting a Mass to be celebrated in his honor at St. Gall Abbey.

75. VENERABLE PAULA RENATA CARBONI
(1908-1927)

UNLIKE many in this volume, who were taught the fundamentals of the Catholic religion by their religious parents, Paula Carboni never heard the family speak of God. But she did learn about the Faith from an aunt, Giuseppina Majeski, who had Paula secretly baptized when the child was very young.

When the family moved to Grottazzolina, Italy, where Paula continued her studies, they lived near a family who were pious Catholics. For the first time, Paula and her sister were enveloped in a Christian atmosphere where they started to know God, to study the catechism and to frequent the parish church. They were instructed by the parish priest, received Holy Communion and were confirmed, all without their father's knowledge. Finally, one day, with "steadiness and sweetness," Paula revealed the secret to her father. Unable to change his daughters' views, he left them to follow a Faith he detested.

Paula made steady progress in virtue, especially after reading *The Story of a Soul*, written by St. Thérèse of Lisieux. She was so taken with the book that she began to imitate the Saint, hoping to become just like her.

At the age of 13, Paula began to suffer from a form of colic that often forced her to bed. She considered the illness as a precious gift of God and even looked for occasions to mortify herself. She wanted to devote herself totally to God and dreamed of becoming a missionary. Her bodily condition would prevent this; instead, she offered herself to God for the conversion of sinners. A few years later she made a total consecration of herself to the love of God by making a vow of virginity on May 21, 1927 when she was 19 years old.

During August of the same year, while enduring a problem with indigestion, Paula contracted typhus, which brought about a very high fever. She remained peaceful and was happy to complete her immolation as a victim to the love of God. She offered her sufferings for the conversion of sinners, but especially for her father, that he would convert to God.

Over the objections of her father, Paula saw her confessor and received the Sacraments. She died a holy death on September 11, 1927. The father did not attend the funeral services in the parish church, but he did accompany the remains to the cemetery. While looking at the casket as it was placed in the grave, he remarked, "Now she is with her God." Paula's prayers for the conversion of her father were answered some years later when he reconciled himself with God and received the Catholic Faith.

The informative process for the beatification of Paula Renata Carboni was begun in 1951. In 1965 her remains were exhumed and entombed in the church of the Madonna of Mercy in Fermo, Italy. Paula was declared Venerable in 1993.

76. Venerable Pauline Marie Jaricot
(1799-1862)

PAULINE was the last of the seven children born to a wealthy silk merchant of Lyons, France. Little is known of her early childhood except that when she was prepared for Holy Communion, Jansenism was then in full force. This was an extremely rigorous spirituality that consumed young minds with the horror of sin and doubts about forgiveness. For years Pauline is said to have haunted confessionals, seeking assurance of God's mercy.

She grew into a young woman of great beauty and grace, which attracted many admirers. She is said to have had a slender figure, dark eyes and dark curls that framed her oval face. She was something of a flirt, attracting male attention and female envy. Pauline herself wrote, "I dressed myself in all my finery, believing myself worthy of universal admiration and preening myself with the conceit of a peacock. Self-love came forcefully into my heart . . . I would have had to be made of ice not to enjoy the flattery, compliments and gentle words of praise I received . . . "

Life for Pauline was beautiful. She had wealth and position; but all that changed for a time in 1814 when Pauline fell from a chair on which she had been standing to reach something on the top shelf of her wardrobe. Although no bones were broken, the remedy employed for the pain she continued to experience was bleeding, which was then a common medical practice. This only produced a general physical deterioration, convulsions, body spasms, loss of weight and erratic speech. Pauline slowly regained her health during an eight-month visit to the family's country estate at Tassin, which was located not far from Lyons.

After Pauline was fully restored to health and was again participating in her former activities, Divine Providence intervened when one day she attended Mass in the Church of St. Nizier. Dressed in one of her more sumptuous outfits, she heard the priest give a scorching homily against vanity. She was greatly affected and afterwards visited the priest, who became her spiritual director. Now only 17 years old, Pauline made a drastic adjustment in her life when she sold her jewelry and distributed the money to the needy. As a sign of her final break with the past, she gave away her beautiful dresses. She clothed herself in a plain purple dress that she disliked and began works of charity. She attended Mass daily, advanced rapidly in virtue and made a vow of perpetual chastity.

Pauline was a born organizer. She gathered together wayward girls into an association named *Reparatrices*—"Women of Reparation"—and gave them a simple rule of life. They had regular meetings, worked at positions that Pauline found for them and assisted the poor and the sick. Pauline began another organization by collecting from workers pennies which would assist the missions. This organization became known as the Society for the Propagation of the Faith. Pauline also founded the Association of the Holy Childhood, by which pennies were collected for the ransoming of pagan babies. Still another organization she founded was that of the Living Rosary, in which 15 members each adopt a Mystery of the Rosary to recite each day.

All her life, since the time of establishing these organizations, Pauline would suffer from criticism, harassment, insults, false rumors and envy. She was also destined to suffer physically from a variety of ailments.

While staying in Rome, she was diagnosed as having a growth on her lung. At this time she met the future St. Madeleine Sophie Barat. Too sick to visit the Pope to speak with him about her organizations, Pauline had the rare privilege of the Pope visiting her in her sickroom. She was again privileged—after being cured at the shrine of the martyr, St. Philomena—when another devotee of St. Philomena, St. Jean Marie Vianney, the famous Curé of Ars, visited her to learn about the cure. For a time he served as Pauline's spiritual director.

Several years after the miraculous cure, Pauline became seriously ill with a congested liver, an infected lung and a bad heart, conditions that would recur throughout the rest of her life. When she was 61 years old, these conditions became quite serious, especially when she suffered from a build-up of body fluids which made her body grow larger and heavier. Doctors held no hope for her recovery. The poor who had benefited from her charity now provided her with food and comfort.

After begging pardon of her companions for her faults, Pauline cried out, "Mary, my Mother, I am all yours!" and died on January 9, 1862. The official opening of her cause for beatification was signed by Pope Pius XI in 1930. She was declared Venerable on February 25, 1963.

77. SAINT PEREGRINE LAZIOSI (1260-1345)

PEREGRINE was the only son of wealthy parents and was born in Forli, Italy. As a young man he led a worldly life and then drifted into politics, joining an anti-papal party. After a popular uprising, the Pope sent as mediator the future St. Philip Benizi, a member of the Servites. As an act of defiance, Peregrine struck Philip Benizi on the face. The holy Servite's reply was to offer the other cheek, an action that brought his assailant to immediate repentance. This is the only known instance in the lives of the Saints in which a future saint accosted another future saint. Peregrine was overwhelmed with apologies and tears, to which St. Philip responded by consoling his penitent, while exhorting him to amend his life and to cultivate a childlike devotion to the Mother of God. Peregrine then turned from his worldly companions and began spending long hours in the chapel of Our Lady in the Cathedral. One day the Blessed Mother appeared to him and encouraged him to go to Siena and enter the Servite Order. Peregrine immediately obeyed, received the Servite habit and was eventually admitted to Holy Orders. He was outstanding for his fervent celebration of the Holy Sacrifice of the Mass, he was eloquent in preaching, and he was untiring in converting and reconciling sinners.

After a time, Peregrine was afflicted with a spreading cancer of the foot that not only brought him excruciating pains, but also made him an object of revulsion to others. He bore his condition without a murmur of complaint. When the doctors advised that only an amputation of the foot would relieve the condition, Peregrine spent the night before the operation in prayer before his crucifix. He then fell into a deep slumber and awoke completely cured, much to the amazement of the doctors, who testified that they could no longer detect any trace of the disease in him. St. Peregrine lived to the age of 85 and died a most holy death in the city of his birth. He is the Patron Saint of cancer sufferers and was canonized in 1726 by Pope Benedict XIII.

78. BLESSED PIERINA MOROSINI (1931-1957)

*P*IERINA was the first child born in her family. Following her came nine brothers. Born on January 7, 1931, Pierina lived a peaceful and prayerful life with her family on a small farm in Fiobbio, which is located in the diocese of Bergamo in northern Italy.

Pierina was a willing assistant to her mother in helping with her brothers and performing her chores. She was also a pious child, and she received the Sacraments at the usual age. When she completed her primary studies, Pierina enrolled in a sewing class and thereafter made clothes for herself and the family. When she was only 15 years old, she began working at a cotton mill in nearby Albino in order to help with the family expenses.

To reach Albino, where she had to report for work at 6:00 in the morning, it was necessary for Pierina to walk through a hilly, forested area. During these walks she recited her morning prayers and prepared herself for the reception of the Holy Eucharist at the earliest Mass offered in the church in Albino. Afterward she reported to work. In years to come she would be remembered by her co-workers as being cheerful and having a sweet temperament, but as being not very talkative. After work, she would walk the same path home and help with the household chores. In addition, Pierina belonged to Catholic Action and worked on behalf of the missions and the diocesan seminary. She also helped in the cleaning of the church.

Pierina had a profound attraction to the religious life, but the needs of her family prevented her from leaving. This she accepted as the will of God.

The only pilgrimage Pierina made in her lifetime was a trip to Rome for the beatification of Maria Goretti on April 27, 1947. Naturally, the topic of Maria's heroic martyrdom was the main topic of conversation. When Pierina was asked what she would do if confronted with the same choice experienced by Maria Goretti, she replied that she would willingly imitate Blessed Maria by dying in defense of purity. Pierina was known to add that she would rather die than commit a sin.

Exactly ten years after the beatification, Pierina had a premonition that she too would suffer martyrdom. And so she did, while on her way home from work on April 4, 1957. It was then that she was confronted on the wooded path by a young man who seized her and dragged her into the brush.

Strange to relate, on the day of Pierina's assault, one of her brothers had a premonition that something would happen to her, and therefore he took the wooded path to meet her after work in order to accompany her safely home. Instead, he found his dying sister on the ground with her clothes in disarray and her long hair matted with blood. Bending over her, he saw that her face was bloody and her breathing was slow and labored. When he touched the left side of her face, his hand was immediately covered with blood and pieces of flesh. A huge and ugly wound covered the left side of her face and head. There were many bloodied handprints in the area and indications that Pierina had fought vigorously against the rapist and even attempted to crawl away. Found nearby in the weeds was a rock covered with blood and bits of flesh. It had apparently been used as a hammer to make the wounds that Pierina suffered in the assault.

Pierina was taken to the hospital, where she was treated; but she lapsed into a coma and died two days later, before she could describe or identify her assailant. She was 26 years old.

The doctors reported that she had been a victim of sexual aggression, to which one of the doctors added, "We have here a new Maria Goretti." On the day after the beatification, the Vatican newspaper, *l'Osservatore Romano* (issue of October 5, 1987), reported that "Her skull was broken and she was raped." Pierina is, nevertheless, designated as "virgin," as well as "martyr."

First buried in the public cemetery, her remains are now found in the parish church of Fiobbio, where many of her devotees pray for her intercession before making a pilgrimage to the place of martyrdom.

Pierina Morosini was beatified on October 4, 1987 in a ceremony attended by her mother, Sara, and her surviving brothers. Pierina has been recommended as a model for working girls and as a model of holy purity.

79. SAINT PIO OF PIETRELCINA (1887-1968)

IN THE small town of Pietrelcina in southern Italy, Padre Pio was born on May 25, 1887 to Grazio Mario Forgione and Maria Giuseppa de Nunzio Forgione. He received the name of Francesco, the name of his little brother who had died in infancy. Other children in the family were an older brother and three younger sisters, all of whom benefited from the influence of religious parents who attended daily Holy Mass, recited a Rosary every night and fasted three days a week in honor of Our Lady of Mount Carmel.

Later in life Padre Pio confided that during his younger years he had conversed with Jesus, the Blessed Mother and his guardian angel and that he had been tormented by the devil. It was during these years, around 1897, when he was ten years old, that Capuchin friars canvassed the countryside seeking donations. Francesco immediately felt called to become one of them.

At the age of 15, in 1903, he received the habit of the Order of Friars Minor Capuchin and the name of Pio, a patron saint of Pietrelcina. A year later he made his first profession, and four years later he pronounced his final vows. Ordination to the priesthood took place when Fra (Brother) Pio was 23. By 1911 Padre Pio was beginning to experience his documented ecstasies. But even before this, in 1910, he had received the stigmata, the wounds of Our Lord's Crucifixion, while praying before a large crucifix.

During the years 1911 to 1916, Padre Pio experienced recurring health problems and was sent home to recuperate. He recovered sufficiently to return to his monastery, but then was called for military duty when World War I began. He served, very unhappily, from August 1917 to March of 1918 before being dismissed. After his discharge, he received the transverberation of the heart—a spiritual gift which was also experienced by a number of other saints, including St. Teresa of Avila. The visible stigmata, the five wounds of Christ, would remain with Padre Pio for the next 50 years, until his death, when they would disappear without leaving a trace.

Upon Padre Pio's return to monastic life, news of this favored priest spread, prompting thousands of pilgrims to travel to Pietrelcina to obtain his counsel and relief for their souls through the Sacrament of Penance. To help these pilgrims, Padre Pio spent 19 hours of each day saying Mass, hearing Confessions and handling correspondence. He usually slept a mere two hours each night.

After a period of restrictions and controversies, Padre Pio continued his rigorous schedule and made plans to build a Home for the Relief of Suffering, a hospital which is still in operation. Padre Pio died on September 23, 1968. His death was followed by expressions of grief from over a hundred thousand people who had gathered for his funeral.

Many mystical favors were granted Padre Pio in addition to the stigmata. The blood of these wounds emitted a fragrant perfume, and he had received the gift of bilocation, the ability to be in two places at the same time. In addition, he could read the hearts of both the sinners and the devout who frequented his confessional. To this should also be added the gift of prophecy.

Not only did the good priest experience intense pain from the wounds of Our Lord, but he also suffered from a variety of ailments. His life of penance and contemplation was often marked by very high fevers that amazed attending physicians, as well as by the nausea and indigestion that he had experienced from his student days.

Padre Pio once confessed to his attending physician: "At intervals for several years, I have been stricken with pains which pierce deeply my intestines; now these intervals are so near each other, and the intensity of my suffering is so atrocious, that especially when I ascend the altar steps I must use extraordinary efforts to keep myself from fainting." The examination that followed revealed a hernia that required an operation. This was performed in the year 1929—without anesthetic, which Padre Pio had refused.

Another operation became necessary when a large tumor or cyst was found in the area of Padre Pio's neck. The operation to remove the tumor and the stitching of the wound took about half an hour. During that operation, which again was performed without an anesthetic, there was not "a word or complaint on the part of the patient." When asked if the tumor ever bothered him, Padre Pio answered, "Certainly I had pain"—all of which he had suffered in silence.

To all that Padre Pio endured during his monastic life, we can add another serious suffering, that of being assaulted on occasion by an angry and vicious devil and then enduring many times the wounds left after these attacks.

Padre Pio's holy life—which included lifelong pain, a monastic life filled with tiring duties, the practice of many virtues, and great love of God and the Blessed Mother—all was recognized when he was beatified in 1999 and canonized on June 16, 2002.

Padre Pio has left us a consoling thought that has encouraged many and could prove beneficial to those who suffer. As he once told a spiritual child: "Pray, hope and don't worry." These words might well console those who experience not only sickness, but also the many other trials endured in the hardships of life.

80. SERVANT OF GOD
RACHELINA AMBROSINI (1925-1941)

NOWN as "the girl who lived for Heaven," Rachelina Ambrosini was born in Venticano, Italy on July 2, 1925 to devout parents, who were careful to instill in her a love of the Faith and a devotion to all that pertained to the Church. She proved to be a docile student with a vivacious nature. During her primary school years, she contracted measles, from which she recovered completely. During these school years she earned the respect and love of the students, teachers, and all who knew her.

In Bari, Italy, she continued her studies at Liceo Cabrini where she distinguished herself as a diligent student and as a ready assistant to all who needed help, especially the poor and the weak. She was noted for her filial respect for the nuns and for her love of the Church and her devout reception of the Sacraments. She was carefully guided in the spiritual life by a priest-uncle and reached the heights of Christian perfection.

When her health began to decline in 1941, she was diagnosed as having purulent otitis, a severe infection of the ear. Untreated for a time, the infection spread, causing a number of serious health concerns, accompanied by severe pain and a threat to her life. Realizing that she would not recover, she predicted the day of her death, and her prediction eventually proved to be correct.

No one actually believed she would die, but after being anointed by the chaplain of the hospital, she received the Blessed Sacrament with transports of joy and gratitude. The chaplain turned to those around the sickbed and said with all seriousness, "She is an angel, not of this earth." Rachelina died on the day she had predicted, March 10, 1941. She was 15 years old.

She was first buried in the local cemetery, but in 1958 her remains were entombed in the parish church of Venticano, where her grave is a place of pilgrimage for devotees, who offer countless prayers for her intercession.

The informative process for Rachelina's beatification was begun by the Archbishop of Benevento and was completed in 1991. The cause for her beatification was accepted by the Congregation for the Causes of Saints in 1995.

81. Saint Rafqa (1832-1914)

AFQA was born in Himlaya, a village of Northern Metn, Lebanon. She was the only child of her mother, Rafqa Gemayel, who died while the child was only six years old. The saint's father, Mourad Saber Shabaq al-Rayes, found it necessary to send Rafqa to work as a maid when she was 11 years old on account of the tension between the child and her stepmother and also because of financial difficulties.

When Rafqa announced at the age of 14 that she felt called to the religious life, her father objected, but at the age of 21 she entered the order of the Marians of the Immaculate Conception. Following her year as a postulant, she was received into the congregation on the feast of St. Joseph, March 19, 1861 and was given the name Sister Mary Anissa (Agnes).

She taught catechism for many years, until a crisis in her congregation found her joining the Lebanese Maronite Order (1871-1914). She was then given a new name in honor of her mother: Sister Rafqa (Rebecca). She spent 26 years in the monastery of St. Simon in observance of the rule, in prayer, silence, sacrifice and austerity.

During the year 1885, on the feast of the Holy Rosary, Sister Rafqa prayed in the monastery church to have some part in the sufferings of Our Lord's Passion. Soon she began experiencing pains in the head which moved to her eyes. All attempts to cure her failed. Then, a visiting American doctor suggested an operation on the afflicted eye. For this, Sister Rafqa refused anesthesia. Sadly, during the course of the surgery her eye became completely detached; soon after, the disease moved to the other eye. Unbearable pain in her head continued for 12 years. During this time Sister Rafqa remained patient and uncomplaining and helped the community by knitting small items. After completely losing her sight in 1907, she became paralyzed due to the dislocation of her right hip and leg.

After many years of intense pain, Rafqa died on March 23, 1914 and was buried in the monastery cemetery. Four days later, miraculous cures through her intercession were being reported. Later, on July 10, 1927, her body was transferred to a shrine in the corner of the monastery chapel.

Pope John Paul II declared Sister Rafqa Venerable in 1982. She was beatified by the same pontiff in 1985 and canonized by him on June 10, 2001.

During the time of the canonical process in 1981, specialists in ophthalmology, neurology and orthopedics concluded that the most likely correct diagnosis of St. Rafqa's illness was tuberculosis with ocular localization and multiple abnormal bony growths.

82. SERVANT OF GOD
RAMON MONTERO NAVARRO (1931-1945)

RAMON was born in Spain at a time when a persecution of the Catholic Faith was gathering momentum. Communist forces were intent on harassing priests and religious, sacred objects were being burned, while churches were either vandalized or destroyed. Because of this confusion, Ramon's First Holy Communion was delayed, but the family continued their usual prayers, gathering each evening for the recitation of the Rosary.

Both of Ramon's parents attended daily Mass. His mother was a devotee of Our Lady of Mount Carmel and the Brown Scapular, and she instilled this devotion in her children.

When Ramon finally received the Eucharist for the first time, his mother asked him if he had requested anything of Our Lord. His answer was astounding: "I asked the Lord to make me like the Beloved Disciple, St. John. Let Him send me suffering, let Him send me whatever He wants. I want to offer myself up for you, for sinners, for everybody. But let Him send me much suffering, so that He lives in me like in His Beloved Disciple."

Ramon had learned about St. John from a Vincentian nun who sometimes visited the family. This good nun talked with Ramon about the sufferings of this disciple, and the boy's comments surprised and pleased her. Afterwards she was to remark, "This is an angel."

The suffering that Ramon had asked for at the time of his First Holy Communion was soon granted at the time the family lived in the country, during the unrest of the Spanish Civil War (1936-1939). The children of the area delighted in taking rides on a mule, but one day the mule reared up, throwing Ramon to the ground. He landed on his back and was speechless for more than half an hour. While his mother massaged his back, she noticed that the vertebrae were not in alignment; she consulted a specialist, who prescribed a corset-like bandage. Soon an abscess developed on his back. The bandage was then exchanged for a plaster cast, which caused other difficulties.

After several open sores appeared, the doctor advised Ramon to lie on his stomach. This caused great discomfort, which he bore without complaint. When five sores developed, Ramon likened them to the five wounds of Our Lord.

The physician soon discovered that Ramon had developed Pott's disease, which causes the destruction of the vertebral bones. The Brothers of St. John of God, who minister to the sick, explained to the parents that the disease is so excruciating that often they had to restrain children, who usually attempted to end their lives due to the excessive pain. This was unnecessary for Ramon, who told his doctors that Jesus was assisting him and that he wanted to accept whatever the Lord sent him.

On days when the pain was almost unbearable, he found some comfort in a picture of Spain's patroness, the *Virgen del Pilar*. He would also ask family members to gather near him to recite the Rosary. At the third decade, Ramon would announce that he felt much relieved.

The development of a kidney stone added to his sufferings. When a doctor prescribed morphine, Ramon refused to accept it and he pleaded with his mother not to force him to take it. He insisted on suffering what the Lord had given him.

The priests of the town knew that Ramon was extraordinary, and they told his story to visiting priests, who as a result went to see the youngster. One priest engaged in conversation with Ramon at such length that he left convinced that Ramon was being enlightened by the Holy Spirit, since the only formal instruction he had received was for his First Holy Communion. Another priest declared, "I've never seen an Angel, but I think that if one did take flesh, he would have to be something like Ramon."

Soon the clergy and laity alike were appealing to Ramon for prayers, with many of the requests being answered with amazing results, as witnessed by several priests.

When Carmelite friars moved into the area, they began to bring Holy Communion to Ramon and supplied him with spiritual reading. Since Ramon dearly loved Our Lady of Mount Carmel, a dispensation was given for Ramon to be clothed in the habit of a Carmelite tertiary. He was taught to pray the Little Office of Our Lady of Mount Carmel and was instructed in the obligations of a Carmelite tertiary.

On the feast day of Our Lady of Mount Carmel, July 16, 1942, Ramon somehow gathered the energy to attend services in the church. Afterward his health began to deteriorate rapidly.

After seeing his mother suffering anxieties about his condition, Ramon told her, "Everything you are suffering on my account, if you will put up with it with patience and joy, you too will earn a very good place in Heaven. The same goes for Dad . . . "

Ramon received the Holy Eucharist for the last time on February 1, 1945. Soon after, as Ramon's eyes were fixed on the crucifix, the church bells rang the midday Angelus. It was then that Ramon peacefully died in his mother's arms. He was 13 years old.

The cause for his beatification has been initiated in his diocese.

83. ROSE PRINCE (1915-1949)

HE preserved body of Rose Prince created great excitement when it was discovered by workmen who were then re-locating graves that were considered to be too close to the Lejac Indian Residential School in British Columbia. The priest and the sisters of the school were notified, and even the children were permitted to view the body. A former student reported, "There was not a spot on her face, not a mark on her. She was such a lovely person. The flowers she was holding had wilted, but she was just lying there, all propped up on her pillow, with a little smile on her face."

Although countless people have visited her tomb after the discovery of her incorrupt body, Father Jules Goulet, who has investigated Rose's cause for beatification, has stated that many were already visiting her grave before the discovery of her bodily preservation.

Rose belonged to an Indian tribe known as the Carrier Nation and was the third of nine children. At the age of seven, Rose began attending the Lejac Residential School, but at the age of nine, tragedy struck. A witness to the accident relates that someone was carrying a large bench and lost control of it, causing it to fall against Rose's back. It is not known if she was examined by doctors, but all suspected that her back had been broken and that this is what caused her almost constant pain thereafter and produced a terrible deformity in her body.

Although suffering, Rose, at the age of nine, was known as a peacemaker between feuding children and was admired for her

205

compassion. One of her friends said that "She was very ill after the accident, but she never complained." Another added that Rose was "quiet, nice, and sensitive to the feelings of others . . . She was special to the sisters and her schoolmates, who looked up to her and respected her." Another said that Rose "was a saint! She had the patience of a saint."

In the opinion of Sister Bridie Dollard, who taught Rose for three years, "Rose was very self-conscious about the painful curvature of the spine . . . yet she was a hard worker and a brilliant student, kind, lovely, gentle and compassionate."

When Rose was 17 years old, her mother died. The father remarried, but this produced a problem for Rose, since she knew her stepmother did not care for her, and probably never would. Rose stayed at the school from then on and eventually graduated. Not wanting to return home, she was accepted as a member of the staff and continued living at the school. She remarked at the time, "I've got family here: our Blessed Mother and her Son, Jesus. They are my parents. I feel so close to them that I don't want to go away."

At school she did secretarial work, as well as cleaning, mending and helping young children. She also painted greeting cards and embroidered flowers on altar cloths and vestments. It is known that she performed her tasks cheerfully. "Rose loved to sing, and always sang or hummed while she was doing her chores. Her fingers were always busy with bead work or crocheting." She was also faithful in her religious exercises, attending Mass daily, and in spite of her pain, she spent many hours kneeling in adoration before the Blessed Sacrament.

When Rose was in her early thirties, she became very ill with tuberculosis and by 1949 she was bedridden. She was hospitalized for a time at Vanderhoof, where she was admired for her patience and serenity. She died peacefully on August 19 after receiving the Holy Eucharist.

The sisters had some difficulty in arranging the body in the casket because of her deformity. After placing a large pillow under her head, they were able to place the body in the proper position. Rose was buried the next day in the Lejac cemetery on her 34th birthday.

Because Rose's preserved body was discovered during the first week of July (two years after burial), this time is observed every year with a three-day pilgrimage which is attended by a large number of devotees, in addition to members of the clergy and the Bishop. Father Jules Goulet has stated that "The people around Fraser Lake have received many, many favors through her intercession."

The inquiry for the cause of her beatification has already begun.

84. Santos Franco Sanchez (1942-1954)

*S*INCE he attended a school conducted by the Carmelite friars, it is not surprising that Santos Sanchez dreamed of entering the minor seminary of that Order. The Carmelite influence was also felt in the family since two of Santos' sisters became cloistered Carmelite nuns and both parents were Carmelite tertiaries.

Santos was born July 6, 1942 at Hinojosa del Duque (Cordoba), Spain. His parents urged their ten children to make frequent visits to the Blessed Sacrament and to love the Blessed Mother of Mount Carmel, to whom the children had been consecrated while they were still in the womb.

Santos was a normal child who joined in the games of his peers and contributed to their noisy and unrestrained play. It was Santos who maintained peace between playmates and invariably took the side of the weaker companion. He was also known for settling disagreements between his brothers and sisters.

Santos' health was excellent until the end of November 1953 when his right ear began to cause pain. When a discharge developed, he was brought to a doctor, who declared it a minor problem. But headaches finally prevented Santos from attending school. When the pain grew worse, he told his mother, "My head hurts a lot, but the doctors say I don't have anything. Don't worry about it, Mom. Let what God wants be done."

During the month of December the condition worsened and a fever came on. Although suffering, Santos showed no signs of irritation or impatience and accepted his condition as God's Will.

Since the doctor refused to accept the seriousness of the boy's condition, the family brought him to another doctor, who offered his opinion that the problem was in the nervous system and prescribed a tranquilizer.

When Santos began experiencing dizzy spells, the father took him to an old friend, a retired doctor, who diagnosed the problem correctly. Santos was suffering from meningitis. Since time had been wasted in making the correct diagnosis, his condition had developed into a fatal one. There was no hope for a cure. The infection had spread to the brain, and little could be done to alleviate the pressure and pain, although the doctor did make an incision behind the boy's ear to drain some of the infected material.

When a priest suggested that his sufferings be offered for the Church and the missions, Santos replied, "From the first moment that I began to experience pain, I haven't stopped offering everything to the Lord for all those intentions . . . and also for sinners." Both the priest and the hospital staff were edified and amazed by the serenity of the young patient.

One day, when Santos was experiencing extreme pain, he was heard to say in a soft voice, "My God, take me to Heaven. I'm too small to suffer so much. However, Your will be done. Everything just as You will it. I offer it to You for sinners, for the missions."

Periodic convulsions racked Santo's poor emaciated body while he writhed in pain. After one of the convulsions, he was lying so still that his family checked his pulse to see if he were still alive. To this Santos assured them: "No, not yet. I still have more to suffer. God only knows when I'll go to Heaven. I offer everything to Him." Another time he was heard to say, "You suffered more than this on the Cross, and when they crowned You with thorns, Your head ached very much."

One of Santos' doctors, who paid him a visit every morning, was a professed atheist. During one visit, when Santos spoke to him about the Blessed Virgin and his guardian angel who gave him strength to suffer, the doctor admitted, "This child has something special about him; if I didn't see him myself, I wouldn't believe it."

Santos died on February 6 after praying, "Take me, take me up to Heaven, my dear Mother . . . God's Will be done." It was the first Saturday of the month, a day dedicated to the Blessed Mother. Santos was 11 years old.

The cause for the eventual beatification of Santos Franco Sanchez has been entrusted to the Carmelite Order.

85. SAINT SERAPHINA (d. 1253)

ORN in San Gimignano, Italy, Seraphina is remembered there as a young girl who accepted great bodily suffering in perfect resignation to the Will of God. She was born into poverty, yet she was known for her charity and for giving her food to those more unfortunate than herself. At a young age, she became proficient in household skills, such as sewing and spinning, and was a wonderful help to her mother.

While Seraphina was still very young, her father died, and it was about this time that this beautiful young girl was attacked by a series of illnesses that left her unattractive and an object of pity. It seemed that all her organs were affected, especially her head, eyes and feet. Soon a paralysis claimed her body.

In offering her sufferings to Our Lord, she refused a soft bed, and instead, she consigned herself to a hard plank. Serphina lay on this board for six years in one position, owing to her paralysis. Constant contact with the wood caused the plank eventually to rot and adhere to her skin, producing unbearable pain.

The devoted mother, reduced after the father's death to abject poverty, was forced periodically to leave the patient while she went begging or looking for work. While the mother was gone, the helpless Seraphina was forced to endure the presence of rats, which occasionally gnawed at her flesh or licked her blood.

In constant pain, Seraphina was nevertheless peaceful, and while gazing upon the crucifix, she was known to repeat numerous times, "Dear Jesus, it is not my wounds that pain me but Thine."

Seraphina had to endure another burden when her mother died, since she was now completely destitute, except for one devoted friend, Beldia. A few neighbors visited her, but they gave her only a little attention, due to their repugnance to her wounds.

Seraphina had a great devotion to Pope St. Gregory the Great, who, she was told, had suffered from various diseases. She prayed fervently to this Saint that she might have patience in her affliction. A few days before her death, the Saint appeared to her and said, "Dear child, on my festival, God will give you rest." On the feast day of St. Gregory the Great, Seraphina died.

It is reported that when her body was removed from the rotten board on which she had lain for so long, the wood was found to be covered with white violets, which gave off a heavenly scent. White violets which bloom in the area about the time of the Saint's feast day are known in her memory as "Santa Fina."

86. BLESSED SERVULUS (d. 590)

HAT we know of Blessed Servulus is given us by none other than St. Gregory the Great. One day, in the Basilica of St. Paul in Rome, St. Gregory was preaching on the Gospel of the day, that being the parable of the sower whose seeds fell on rocks, thorns or good ground. "But that [seed] on the good ground, are they who in a good and perfect heart, hearing the word, keep it, and bring forth fruit in patience." (*Luke* 8:15). To illustrate the parable, St. Gregory told the story of Servulus, a holy invalid who begged near the Church of St. Clement. Many in St. Gregory's congregation had seen or known the holy beggar. St. Gregory has also told of Blessed Servulus in Book IV of his *Dialogues.*

Blessed Servulus, St. Gregory relates, had suffered all his life from palsy. Such was the violent shaking of the body and the uncontrolled movements of his muscles that "he could not stand, nor sit up in his bed, neither was he ever able to put his hand into his mouth or to turn from one side to the other. His mother and brethren did serve and attend him, and what he got in alms, by their hands he bestowed upon other poor people."

St. Gregory continues that Servulus could not read, but he somehow acquired a copy of the Scriptures and had religious men read it to him. "Yet did he fully learn the Holy Scripture and he was careful in his sickness always to give God thanks, and day and night to praise His Holy Name."

St. Gregory says, "When the time was come in which God determined to reward this, his great patience, the pain of his

213

body struck inwardly to his heart, which he feeling, and knowing that his last hour was not far off, called for all who lodged in his house, desiring them to sing hymns." But he soon asked for silence, saying, "Do ye not hear the great and wonderful music which is in Heaven?" At the time of his death, those present experienced a sweet fragrance that did not dissipate until after the time of his burial.

The following comment is given by St. Gregory the Great: "The memory of this poor, sick beggar condemns those who, when blessed with good health and fortune, neither do good works nor suffer the least cross with noteworthy patience."

87. Servant of God Silvio Dissegna
(1967-1979)

ILVIO was born in Turin, Italy to an outstanding couple who fostered in him a deep love of the Faith. From his earliest years, Silvio demonstrated a lively intelligence and a love of all activities that were normal for his age. He was healthy and vivacious and liked to play ball, to ride on his bicycle, and to watch television cartoons. He was a popular boy who was known for always having a pleasant smile. He was also known for having a close relationship with Jesus. He was heard to say, "I want my actions to be good. I want to pray with joy and to help those in need, respecting all."

At the beginning of the year 1978, Silvio experienced the first symptoms of a serious illness. A persistent pain in his left leg resulted in several visits to his doctor, who prescribed certain medications. When the pain became intense, various tests were made regarding his condition, which resulted in a diagnosis of bone cancer. When the father heard the sad report, he was extremely distressed, but Silvio encouraged him, saying: "Papa, have courage. Jesus will not abandon us. Papa, I will pray for you. I also need Jesus in order to be brave." To his worried mother, Silvio remarked, "If I die, it is not important. I will suffer to the end. Mother, we will be happy and content only in Paradise."

It was evident that Silvio was guided by the Holy Spirit. He often remarked, "Today, I offer my suffering for the Pope and the Church." Another day he would say, "Today, I offer for the clergymen." And again, "Today, I offer my pains for the conversion of sinners." Another time, his pains were offered for the missions and for missionaries.

For a time, Silvio continued his studies at home, until prescribed medical procedures needed to be started, especially chemotherapy.

Every day Silvio asked to receive the Holy Eucharist, and he was serene in his suffering. During his most painful days, he would remark, "My vocation is to suffer . . . I offer my pains with those of Jesus Crucified, for the entire world . . . I must remain with Jesus, the one I have in my heart. Jesus, I suffer like You when You were crucified . . . I am covering the road to Calvary, and afterward there will be the crucifixion . . . Jesus wants from me many sufferings and prayers."

The cancer that had first affected Silvio's leg coursed through his body, so that his sight was lost in June and his hearing in September. Many nights were spent in extreme pain; still, the young patient was able to recite the Fifteen Mysteries of the Rosary and always looked forward to the next day's reception of the Eucharist.

After receiving the Anointing of the Sick, Silvio died on September 24, 1979 with an angelic smile on his face. He was 12 years old. His funeral was held in the parish church of Poirino, where it was estimated that 40 or more priests attended.

Silvio's sanctity was quickly recognized by diocesan officials, who opened the cause for his beatification the next February. The diocesan process ended in October 2001 when the official documents were given to the Congregation for the Causes of Saints.

Two biographies of Silvio soon came out. When Cardinal Peter Palazzini, Prefect of the Congregation for the Causes of Saints, read one of them, he wrote: "The example of Silvio illustrates that children are able to attain heroic virtues and are worthy of canonization."

Pope John Paul II, after reading the documents relative to the cause, exclaimed: "Silvio is a beautiful example of an innocent soul who willingly endured pain for the love of God. We entrust his cause to the Madonna."

88. VENERABLE STEPHEN KASZAP
(1916-1935)

ORN in Hungary in 1916, Stephen admitted that as a young child he was obstinate, aggressive and had a bad temper, even to the point of throwing objects when irritated or teased by his four siblings. On the other hand, he could be happy and was co-operative in performing daily chores. While attending school conducted by Cistercian monks, he took part in so many high-spirited antics and so much student mischief that he revealed in his journal: "In general, I was quite willful and sometimes worked around the rules, but I was not perverted or corrupt. I have no doubt at all that I often irritated and annoyed the teachers . . . " Gradually the influence of the monks changed Stephen's character, so that he began to make spiritual progress. He served Holy Mass and noted, "I shall serve every day that I can." He joined the Congregation of Mary, whose main purpose was to increase the devotion to and love of the Blessed Mother and to spread devotion to her. He was a member of the Boy Scouts, and, according to his patrol leader, he carried out orders without complaint or excuse. "I could always trust him completely and always count on his support."

Stephen loved the outdoors and often got up early in the morning to go to the edge of the forest to pray, "where everything speaks about our Almighty Creator." Yet he was always on time for morning Mass. He had many interests, including musical compositions, and composers such as Mozart and Verdi. He studied French, Italian and Spanish, and he became so adept that he was able to serve as translator for Italian students visiting Hungary. Stephen was also a champion gymnast and student vice-president. After graduating from school at 18 years of age, he entered the Jesuit novitiate at the Hungarian Manresa House on July 30, 1934. He was filled with enthusiasm and happiness and was determined to increase in virtue and love of God.

Stephen began his novitiate in excellent health, but soon he became hoarse and lost his voice. His tonsils needed medical attention, and then, soon after Christmas, his ankles became swollen with arthritic pains, so that he could barely walk. Abscesses formed on his fingers, then on his neck and face. Later, they also developed on his thighs and loins, and his fever rose to alarming heights. His torments must have been severe since he wrote in his journal, "Any cross God gives must be carried with joy . . . I suffer gladly for Christ, and I don't run from pain."

In addition to these sufferings, he was diagnosed with pleurisy and he endured serious nosebleeds, which were so severe that they were nearly fatal. It soon became necessary for the bleeding vein to be cauterized. The operation was scheduled for March 19, the feast of St. Joseph. After the operation, Stephen whispered to his novice master, "Holy Communion helped me greatly today, and that is why I was so calm going in for surgery. I trust St. Joseph very much. How small our sufferings are and how much the Church needs them. These thoughts make suffering much easier for me."

As soon as he could leave his bed, Stephen began to help his fellow patients and apparently spoke to them about the blessings of receiving Holy Communion. His influence was most noticeable at the Easter Holy Communion, when ten out of the eleven patients in his hospital ward received Our Lord well prepared and with deep faith. The 11th patient, a non-Catholic, exclaimed, "I never thought there was so much faith, harmony and love in the Catholic Faith."

For a time Stephen's condition improved, so that he resumed his studies for the priesthood, but it became apparent that he did not have the required health to continue. With the assurance that he could return when his health improved, Stephen left the novitiate with a heavy heart and a sad farewell. He wrote in his journal: "Bodily sufferings cannot be compared to those of the soul. My whole life should be a continuous yes to God."

He was home only a few days when he was again admitted to the hospital, where he was diagnosed with erysipelas. After two weeks, he returned home and continued the schedule of prayer and study he had practiced in the novitiate.

Weeks later, he returned to the hospital for the removal of his tonsils, which caused several hemorrhages and the failure of the incision to heal properly. In just a few days he was diagnosed with a tumor in the throat that caused such difficulty in breathing that every breath was increasingly painful and desperate. Unable to speak, Stephen communicated by writing on a pad, asking for what was needed. What he asked for most was for a priest to visit and administer the Last Sacraments.

Since the nurse did not suspect that he was dying, the priest was not notified, so that Stephen died without the consolation of the Church from the Last Rites. After his death, however, the priest did visit and administer Extreme Unction—which can be administered for a few hours after apparent death, according to the discretion of the priest—plus the priest gave the papal blessing. After Stephen's death, this last notation was found in his journal: "God be with you! We will meet in Heaven! Do not weep; this is my birthday in Heaven. God bless you all!"

Stephen was only 19 years old. Seven years later, the Bishop, Msgr. Lajos Shvoy, initiated the cause for his beatification. The remains of Stephen Kaszap were carried in a triumphal procession in 1942 to his present resting place in a chapel of the Prohaszka Memorial Church. Since then, many have appealed for his intercession, and many cures have been effected as a result.

Stephen Kaszap's heroic virtues were recognized by Rome in 2006.

89. SAINT SYNCLETICA (d. 400)

O F WEALTHY Macedonian parents, Syncletica was born in Alexandria, Egypt and was inclined toward virtue from childhood. Several suitors were attracted to her great beauty and wealth, but she rejected all proposals of marriage because of the vow of virginity she had made in her youth. At the death of her parents, she and her sister, who was blind, were left heirs to a huge fortune. Syncletica distributed her fortune among the poor, and with her sister, she retired to an unused sepulchral chamber on the estate of a relative. Here, in the presence of a priest, she renewed her consecration to God and cut off her hair as a sign that she renounced the world. Her chief occupations from then on were mortification and prayer.

When Syncletica's virtue became known, many women came to ask her advice about temporal and spiritual matters. With humility, she encouraged them in their trials and urged them along the way of holiness.

The devil, it seems, was quite aware of the good Syncletica was accomplishing and retaliated by tormenting her in so many ways that she was considered another Job.

In the 80th year of her life, she was seized with an intense fever that did considerable damage to her lungs. At the same time, a cancer developed in her mouth. This not only devoured the flesh in that area, but it also afflicted the jaw and the larynx, robbing her of speech. With incredible patience and resignation to God's holy Will, she permitted physicians to pare away from her face the parts that were already dead. Because of these procedures and her frightful condition, she found no rest for the last three months of her life.

When the hour came for her death, Syncletica was surrounded by a heavenly light and was favored with consoling visions. She was 84 years old.

We know of St. Syncletica from various writings, especially that of St. John Climacus, who was apparently familiar with her life.

90. SAINT TERESA OF AVILA (1515-1582)

THROUGHOUT her lifetime, from her youth to her death, Teresa was beset by troubling illnesses which, despite their repeated recurrence, did not interfere with her capacity for intellectual and organizational work or with her spiritual advancement.

Born into a wealthy Catholic family on March 28, 1515, one of ten children, Teresa would be known throughout her life as a beautiful and graceful lady whose charm was undeniable. It is reported that she maintained this charm until the time of her death.

This great reformer of the Carmelite Order was known for her great piety as a child; however, during her adolescence her fervor languished when she became attracted to the romantic, chivalrous literature of her day. After reading religious works given to her by a devout uncle, especially *The Third Spiritual Alphabet* (a work that is still available), she began to reclaim the devotion she had formerly experienced.

When she decided upon a religious vocation, her father at first refused. However, Teresa found a way and entered the Carmelite convent of the Incarnation in Avila, where she took vows in 1536. Two years after entering, her health declined to such a startling degree that her father removed her from the convent for treatment. Teresa writes in her *Autobiography,* "For two months my life was nearly worn out; and the severity of the pain in the heart was very keen. It seemed to me . . . as if it had been seized by sharp teeth. So great was the torment that it was feared it might end in madness . . ."

In addition to the pains in her heart, Teresa also experienced in 1539 what she called "fainting-fits" (catalepsy), which became frequent. These, together with the heart pains, were so serious "that everyone who saw me was alarmed."

For more than eight months Teresa suffered from heart pains and other complications. One night the sickness became so acute that she became insensible and remained in a coma for four days. In fact, many thought she was dead, and a grave was even prepared for her. But Teresa recovered, although she suffered greatly, according to a detailed description of her infirmities in her *Autobiography.* She wrote: "I was bent together like a coil of rope . . . unable to move either arm or foot, or hand, or head, any more than if I had been dead. . . . It is impossible to describe my extreme weakness, for I was nothing but bones. I remained in this state more than eight months, and was paralytic, though getting better for about three years."

Teresa also revealed: "I have been suffering for twenty years from nausea every morning, so that I cannot take any food till past midday, and even occasionally not till later. . . at night before I lie down to rest, that sickness occurs, and with greater pain, for I have to bring it on (vomiting) with a feather or other means. If I do not bring it on I suffer more; and thus I am never free from great pain, which is sometimes very acute, especially about the heart, though the "fainting-fits" are now of rare occurrence. I am also, these eight years past, free from the paralysis and from other infirmities of fever which I had so often."

When Teresa entered the Order, the Rule had been relaxed to such a degree that the speak room was always busy with visitors. Also, royal ladies without vows, accompanied by their servants, lived with the nuns for various periods of time. There were also other practices which were contrary to the original Rule given to the Order by St. Albert of Jerusalem (c. 1149-1214).

After living in these comfortable surroundings for many years, Teresa felt the need to return the Order to its previous, eremitical spirit. She founded the first convent of the reformed or "Discalced" Carmelites in 1562 amid countless persecutions and difficulties. St. John of the Cross, who became a Discalced Carmelite friar, helped to extend the reform to like-minded friars. Thus developed the division between the Carmelite Order of the Ancient Observance (O. Carm.) and the Discalced Carmelite Order (O.C.D.).

Under the rigorous interpretation of the Rule, Teresa attained great heights of mysticism, experiencing mystical phenomena while also founding 17 convents of the reform. In addition, the saint wrote such spiritual classics as *The Way of Perfection, The Interior Castle* and her *Autobiography,* among several other works.

While founding convents throughout Spain and writing these books, St. Teresa suffered recurrent illnesses and severe headaches, as she wrote toward the end of her *Autobiography:* "When I began my prayer that day, my headache was so violent that I thought I could not possibly go on."

On the day before Christmas in the year 1577, Teresa fell and broke her arm. The arm was slow in healing and troubled her for years, due to being incorrectly set. Through the rest of her life the arm continued to cause pain; it actually maimed her so that she needed assistance to dress and undress. Despite the pain and all the difficulties it entailed, she continued her writings and the countless travels she undertook to the 17 convents she had founded throughout Spain.

It has been reported that the saint suffered a paralytic stroke in March of 1580 and then another the same year in August. This was two years before her death. She died in 1582.

St. Teresa of Avila was canonized in 1622 by Pope Gregory XV. Centuries later, she was privileged to be proclaimed the first woman Doctor of the Church. Pope Paul VI conferred this title upon her on September 27, 1970.

91. SAINT THEOPHANES (d. 817)

T. THEOPHANES' father was the governor of the Isles of the Archipelago and died when Theophanes was a mere three years old. After his father's death, Theophanes was heir to a large estate and was placed in the care of Emperor Constantine Copronymus, who had embraced the heresy known as Iconoclasm, which opposed the use of religious images. Under the care of a court official who was a devout Catholic, Theophanes was preserved from the heresy and began to consider a religious vocation.

Upon reaching the proper age, he was forced to marry, but both he and his wife decided to live in perpetual celibacy. His wife later entered religious life. Theophanes retired from the world and erected two monasteries. In one of these, he lived for six years in continual mortification and prayer. Eventually, he was made Abbot of Mount Sigriana, one his foundations.

Theophanes was invited to take part in the Second Council of Nicea, which took place in 787. During this Council, the use and veneration of sacred images was declared a legitimate practice and their use sanctioned. The Fathers of that Council declared that "whether the images were carved or painted, or in whatever material they were wrought, [the sentiment they engendered] was directed to Our Lord, the Blessed Virgin Mary, and the Saints whom they represented." It was therefore enacted that "sacred images were to be restored on the walls of churches, on vestments, on the holy vessels, as well as in private houses and public squares."

This ruling was thereafter observed during the reign of Emperor Constantine Copronymus, but when Leo, the Armenian, ascended the throne in 814, he reversed the policy of his predecessors and tried by all means to suppress the use of images. Realizing the widespread reputation of St. Theophanes, Emperor Leo thought to persuade him to his point of view. If he could win over the Saint, countless others would follow. The Saint, by that time, was suffering from a kidney stone and other painful internal problems which kept him in a perpetual state of extreme pain.

Leo sent Theophanes a document in which he first flattered the Saint, but then wrote: "If you refuse to comply with my desires in this matter, you will incur my utmost displeasure and bring misery and disgrace upon yourself and upon the members of your community." Theophanes responded: "If you think to frighten me into compliance by your threats, as a child is awed by the rod, you are only losing your pains. For although unable to walk, and subject to many other corporal infirmities, I trust in Christ that He will enable me to undergo, in defense of His cause, the sharpest tortures that you can inflict upon my feeble frame."

The Emperor responded by having Theophanes scourged and imprisoned. After receiving 300 stripes with the whip, he was confined for two years in a small and unhealthy dungeon. He was at last removed and banished to the Island of Samothrace, where he died on March 12, 17 days after his arrival, as the result of the treatment he had endured.

92. Servant of God Toni Zweifel
(1938-1989)

ONI Zweifel was born in the historic city of Verona to a family that was financially secure. He attended school in Verona, but when he was 19, he moved to Zurich to study mechanical engineering, remaining at his studies for five years.

When he realized that he could live a Christian vocation through his work, not in addition to it or in spite of it, he began to find Christ in everyday life, especially in his professional work. He became cheerful, whereas before he had possessed a rather serious demeanor. His spiritual life grew deeper with daily Mass, times for mental prayer, and the reading of the Gospels and the classics of spiritual literature.

Toni began his first professional job with a firm in Zurich in 1962. Two years later, he was performing scientific work at the Institute for Thermodynamics. Always a devout Catholic, Toni discovered a closer relationship with God through his scientific and technical work. He developed a number of patents that represented the cutting edge of technology for several decades and earned considerable respect and admiration from his colleagues.

After eight years of working for the Federal Technical Institute, Toni resigned to work entirely for the benefit of the underprivileged. He co-founded and became director of an organization that now supports hundreds of projects in more than 30 countries around the world.

When Toni was 48 years old, he was diagnosed with

leukemia. He underwent several weeks of chemotherapy, and for the next three years he suffered from recurrences.

Understanding that he had almost no chance of survival, Toni accepted the treatments and discomforts with composure and with good humor and was a model patient. He realized that he had been given the opportunity to share in the cross of Christ, and he prepared himself for his eventual meeting with God. He once pointed out to his visiting friends, "If leukemia were more painful than crucifixion, Jesus Christ would have died from leukemia." Toni's friends always left his bedside enriched and strengthened in their faith and in their love of God.

Toni died on November 24, 1989, strengthened by the Sacraments of the Church. The cause for his beatification has been initiated with the appointment of a postulator.

93. WIERA (IDA) FRANCIA (1898-1928)

IERA was a complex person who worried about a great many things. Even as a child she was not the playful, typically happy, outgoing youngster. She was a quiet and prayerful child who recognized her faults and seems to have been always mindful of them. Early on, she was not always a pleasant person, since she often corrected her older sisters and used brusque words. She was also headstrong, preferring her own way rather than what her parents wanted. Those who knew her as a child never imagined that she would struggle to such a degree against what she called her limitations and faults, and attain such an advanced measure of virtue, as to be promoted for the honors of the altar.

Wiera had three sisters and a brother who all lived with their parents and paternal grandparents in the same house. One can only imagine the difficulties that arose with so many personalities under the same roof, especially with a difficult child in their midst.

Wiera was taught by the Sisters of St. Dorothy during her elementary studies, but for high school she attended the public school, where she excelled in her studies to such an extent that at graduation she received a number of scholarships. She left home at the age of 18 to attend the University of Bologna, where she felt very much alone. She had difficulty making friends but was ever ready to help students who were having difficulty with their studies.

It seems that Wiera was always finding fault with herself. She wrote in her diary: "Above all, I'm so cold in religious matters, so un-mortified, so impatient! Today I would have preferred not to go to church because it bores me to go, and to remain there annoys me. How horrible I am, cold, cold, evil . . ." Even so, Wiera continued her religious practices.

One of her biographers wrote: "Wiera is a realist. She details her failings: she is too critical, she uses improper language, she is envious, easily discouraged, irascible to the point of crying out of anger without knowing why, she is proud with a subtle pride which hankers after praise even while refusing it, which refuses to bend down and ask for help, which looks down on the person who doesn't care for her, all the while giving the impression of humility. Wiera is ruthless in her self-analysis because she knows that this is how the Lord sees her."

Wiera received her degree in 1920 and a doctorate the following year, but she felt inadequate and had to force herself to teach. Almost as an answer to prayer, she won a position teaching mathematics and physics in Lecce, which brought her into contact with a gifted spiritual director.

Wiera had problems during her teaching career. She was always anxious about her work, especially at exam time, when she was tormented about giving each student a just and fair evaluation—a hard thing to do since she had over 300 pupils. When her students did not seem interested, she suffered. She also occasionally had disciplinary problems, which she spiritualized by remembering the trials of Our Lord.

In addition to teaching, Wiera participated in the works of Catholic Action. She did this out of a sense of duty, since she felt a certain repugnance to some of the activities that did not appeal to her. But she wanted to do as much good as she could for as many people as she could. She also gave conferences, prepared outlines, encouraged, inspired and exhorted, reminding the members that "we have no right to neglect a single person regardless of how distasteful to us contact with him might be. Jesus loves him and died for him. . . . in any circumstance look at Jesus, see how He acted."

Around this time Wiera listed some of her faults in her diary. She admitted to being "bitter, over-sensitive, intolerant, harsh, moody, impatient, bad-humored, self-centered . . ." She then declared, "I should conquer myself. I wish I could, but I do not always succeed. I suffer a lot because of it. . . ." Still she continued praying and striving to change.

Wiera came in contact with the Carmelite Order and soon became a Third Order member, or tertiary. The rule of the Carmelites gave her the needed order and organization that appealed to a teacher of math. She wore the scapular, recited the Little Office of Our Lady, attended daily Mass, received the Eucharist, meditated, read spiritual books, visited the Blessed Sacrament and examined her conscience. All of this, together with the help of her spiritual director, gave her the strength to war against her imperfections.

We are told by her spiritual director that her thanksgivings after Holy Communion were "protracted, with her head in hands. . . . She was oblivious to all else around her."

Wiera never married, and she knew the religious life was not for her; instead, she made a private vow of perpetual virginity. She regarded this act, made after Holy Communion, as her nuptials, and thereafter she felt obliged to follow her Beloved wherever He went and to do whatever He asked of her.

Wiera was never a physically strong woman. Not helping her health were her constant struggles at self-control and at overcoming her faults, so that she eventually experienced physical exhaustion and bouts of amnesia. Wiera apparently had some kind of intestinal problem, since the doctors operated in 1928.

Her condition became serious when her intestine was perforated. Wiera recognized this as an indication of the end.

She was anointed and received Holy Communion, and after consoling her family and friends, she died on May 28, 1928 at the age of 30.

In her diary she gives some profound advice: "Your sanctification is the first activity to which Jesus wishes you to apply yourself. . . . Holiness is not heroism for a moment, nor even a series of properly so-called heroic acts. . . . Thus every day, or rather every instant, should contribute to form the building of your holiness. . . . Think of being a saint today and begin this very hour, or rather, this minute, and afterward let Jesus act."

It is reported that the diocesan authorities will soon begin an investigation into Wiera Francia's life with a view of submitting a cause to the Congregation for the Causes of Saints for her possible eventual beatification.

94. BLESSED ZELIE GUERIN MARTIN
(1831-1877)

THIS outstanding mother had one daughter who became a Visitation nun and four daughters who became Discalced Carmelite nuns. One of these was the world-renowned St. Thérèse of the Child Jesus and of the Holy Face. The mother did not see any of her daughters enter religious life, since she died at the age of almost 46, before the girls were old enough to realize their vocations.

Zelie Guerin was born on December 23, 1831 at St. Denis-sur-Sarthon near Alencon, France and was baptized on Christmas Eve. A sister, Marie Louise, was born two years previously and a brother, Isidore, was born ten years later.

By her own account, Zelie did not have a happy childhood. Her mother was very austere in her treatment of her two daughters and did not show affection to them. The father was strict too, but he showed them more kindness. Zelie was later to write that her youth was as "sad as a winding-sheet."

At the age of 13, together with her sister, she attended the School of Perpetual Adoration as a day pupil. There, she displayed a keen intelligence and repeatedly won first place for style and composition in her French essays. During these years, Zelie suffered severe headaches as well as respiratory problems, and it was because of her delicate health that the Sisters of Charity of St. Vincent de Paul would not accept her as a postulant when she applied to join them.

Her sister, Marie Louise, entered the Visitation Convent at

Le Mans at the age of 29, and her brother, Isidore, studied medicine in Paris and became a pharmacist.

Once disappointed at not being accepted into religious life, Zelie turned to the Blessed Mother and heard an interior voice which said, "Make Point d'Alencon lace." Zelie went to a professional school to learn the trade. She quickly excelled and left to start her own business.

One day when she was crossing the Bridge of St. Leonard, Zelie noticed a man passing by and again heard that interior voice. It said, "This is he whom I have prepared for you." The man was Louis Martin. Louis' mother had noticed Zelie at the lace-making school and introduced them. Louis and Zelie were married in 1858 and lived in celibacy for ten months, until their confessor convinced them that God intended them to have children. They were blessed with nine children in 13 years, four of whom died in infancy or early childhood.

Zelie had always wanted a son who would someday become a priest. She gave birth to two boys, but both died very young. She was blessed with five daughters who lived past childhood: Marie, Pauline, Leonie, Celine, and her last child, Thérèse—all of whom remembered Zelie as a most loving and caring mother. Thérèse was only four and a half years old at her mother's death, but she was to write, "God granted me the favor of opening my intelligence at an early age and of imprinting childhood recollections deeply on my memory. Jesus in His love willed, perhaps, that I know the matchless mother He had given me but whom His hand hastened to crown in Heaven."

During these childbearing years, while Zelie was overseeing 15 women in her lace-making business, she was also attending to her housekeeping and attending Mass every morning with her husband. She was known for her strong faith, incredible energy and great capacity for work. She was also known as being vivacious and witty, as well as an astute business-woman and a loving and tender mother.

Also during these childbearing years, Zelie was to write to her brother in April 1865, "You know that when I was a girl, I received a blow in the breast, through striking the corner of a table. No notice was taken of it then, but I now have a glandular swelling in the breast which makes me anxious, especially since it has begun to be a little painful . . . It is not that I would shrink from an operation. I am quite ready to undergo it, but I have not full confidence in the doctors here . . . " It should be mentioned here that Zelie did not nurse most of her children, but sent them to a wet nurse.

It is unknown why the operation was delayed and the condition not mentioned until several years later. But then the loving Martin family became very concerned when in October 1876 the swelling in Zelie's breast increased and became so painful that she found it necessary to consult a doctor. The examination revealed a tumor in an advanced stage. Zelie knew there was no hope of recovery, but at the insistence of her brother she consulted a surgeon who was a friend of his. The surgeon only confirmed that it was too late for a surgical procedure.

Although the future looked grim, Zelie's faith was unshaken, and she insisted that God could do with her what He pleased. She was resigned to co-operating with His divine will.

Zelie's condition proved to be most painful at night, and sleep was difficult. In addition, a ganglion on her neck began to swell, causing additional pain. After a time she could not dress herself and relied on Marie to help her. She continued attending Mass in the morning with her husband, but eventually her weakness was so great that she reluctantly remained at home.

She was to write to her brother, "The disease is becoming worse day by day. The arm on the sore side is almost paralyzed, but my hand and fingers can still hold a needle. Besides, I feel sore, as it were, all over, due to a constant fever for the past two weeks. I cannot stand upright anymore, and must remain seated . . . These are for me days of salvation which will never return, and I wish to profit from them. Thus I shall have double profit: I shall suffer less by being resigned, and I shall put in part of my Purgatory while here on earth. I beseech you to ask for me both resignation and patience . . . "

Eventually the tumor began to discharge, and then intestinal troubles and fever presented additional problems. Days later, when a hemorrhage developed, accompanied by a loss of Zelie's voice, her brother's family was summoned. On Tuesday, August 28, 1877 at 12:30 a.m. Zelie died. The following day, she was buried in the family tomb near her four little ones who had preceded her in death. Much later, after the death of Louis Martin, Zelie's brother, Isidore Guerin, had the family grave moved to Lisieux.

The cause for the beatification of Zelie and Louis Martin was initiated in 1957. They were both declared Venerable on March 26, 1994.

On October 19, 2008 both parents of St. Thérèse were beatified in Lisieux by José Cardinal Saraiva Martins, the legate of Pope Benedict XVI.

INDEX OF AILMENTS
AND OTHER PHYSICAL PROBLEMS

E OFFER apologies to the following Saints for exposing their personal problems in this book. However, it is our firm belief that they would willingly expose their problems themselves if they were given the opportunity to help just one suffering patient. With this in mind, we present their afflictions in the hope that their example in times of affliction, and their confidence in the Will of God, will help many in our time to accept fully their own condition, while trusting in a benevolent God.

Continued . . .

Continued . . .

Continued . . .

Continued . . .

BIBLIOGRAPHY*

Agli Amici di Silvio Dissegna, Morto di Cancro a 12 Anni. Special Issue for the Diocesan Process. Edito dall'Associazione "Amici di Silvio." Turin, Italy. 2002.

Amati, Giordano, Bruno Benini, Valentino Maraldi. *Angelina Docile Allo Spirito.* Stilgraf di Cesena. 1998.

Amati, Giordano, Bruno Benini, Mario Morigi, Angelo Pirini. *Prendere Il Largo . . . Con Angelina.* Stilgraf di Cesena. 2002.

Anfrosina Berardi, Serva di Dio. Paper.

Bechard, Henri. *Blessed Kateri Tekakwitha.* The Kateri Center. Caughnawaga, P. Q., Canada. No date.

Benedictine Nun of Stanbrook Abbey, A. *Anne: The Life of Venerable Anne de Guigne.* TAN Books and Publishers, Inc. Rockford, Illinois. 1997.

Bibliotheca Sanctorum. 14 volumes. Citta' Nuova Editrice. Rome, Italy. 1963-2000.

Bibliotheca Sanctorum, Prima Appendice. Citta' Nuova Editrice. Rome, Italy. 1987.

Boday, S.J., Jeno. *Stephen Kaszap, Servant of God.* Paper.

———*Stephen Kaszap, Servant of God.* Our Lady of Hungary Church. Montreal, Quebec, Canada. No date.

Brown, Ann. *No Greater Love: Bl. Gianna: Physician, Mother, Martyr.* New Hope Publications. New Hope, Kentucky. 1999.

Buehrle, Marie Cecilia. *Kateri of the Mohawks.* All Saints Press, Inc. New York. 1954.

Butler, Alban; Herbert Thurston, S.J.; Donald Attwater. *The Lives of the Saints.* 12 Volumes. P. J. Kenedy & Sons. New York. 1934.

Cortesi, Passionista, P. Fulenzio. *La Serva di Dio Mamma Elisabetta, Elisabetta Tasca Serena.* Postulazione Generale Missionari Passionisti. Rome, Italy. 1991.

Cruz, Joan Carroll. *Saintly Men of Modern Times.* Our Sunday Visitor, Inc. Huntington, Indiana. 2003.

———*Saintly Women of Modern Times.* Our Sunday Visitor,

---

* The author regrets that this bibliography is not as complete as it might be. The book *Saints for the Sick* was largely written prior to 2005, but the bibliography had not been finished when Hurricane Katrina destroyed the Cruz home, including the author's reference library, in August of that year.

Inc. Huntington, Indiana. 2004.

———*Saintly Children and Teens of Modern Times.* Our Sunday Visitor, Inc. Huntington, Indiana. 2006.

———*Secular Saints.* TAN Books and Publishers, Inc. Rockford, Illinois. 1989.

Cunningham, Joseph W. *Blessed Gianna Molla.* Immaculata Magazine. Libertyville, Illinois. July/August, 1998.

Da Riese Pio X, Fernando. *For the Love of Life: Gianna Beretta Molla, Doctor and Mother.* 1981.

Decretum Lucen. Canonizationis Servae Dei Anitae Cantieri. Rome, Italy. 1991.

De Giorgi, Salvatore. *Il Vangelo Dei Bambini.* Editrice. Rome, Italy. 1955.

Dolan, O.Carm., Albert H. *Matt Talbot, Alcoholic.* The Carmelite Press. Englewood, New Jersey. 1947.

Dollen, Father Charles. *Charity without Frontiers: The Life-Work of Marie Pauline Jaricot.* The Liturgical Press. Collegeville, Minnesota. 1972.

Giardi, S.C.J., P. Giuseppe. *Antonietta Meo accanto alla croce.* Apostolato della Riparazione. Bologna, Italy. 1962.

Huysmans, J. K. *Saint Lydwine of Schiedam.* TAN Books and Publishers, Inc. Rockford, Illinois. 1979.

Lanzoni, Rev. Riccardo. *Nilde Guerra, Scritti.* Tipografia Faentina. Faenza. 1988.

Lorena D'Alessandro, *Una giovinezza offerta a Dio.* Leaflet. Fabriano, Italy. 1964.

Luigi Rocchi, Un Santo in Carrozzella. Comitato Promotore della Causa di Beatificazione. Tolentino, Italy. 1991.

Maraldi, Valentino. *Angelina, La Sua Vita E L'Eucaristia.* Pamphlet.

Maria Carmelina Leone E Venerabile. Leaflet. Palermo, Italy.

Marion, Francis. *New African Saints.* Ancora Publishers. Milan, Italy. 1964.

Mondrone, S.J., Domenico. *Angiolino, Un Ragazzo Che Seppe Soffrire.* Centro Volontari Della Sofferenza. Rome, Italy. 1992.

Moscone, Felice. *Angiolino Bonetta, Sono tutto della Madonna: dalla testa ai piedi.* C.V. S. Rome, Italy. 1998.

Myriam de G. *Fiaccola Romana, Antonietta Meo (Nennolina).* Roberto Berruti a.c. Turin, Italy. No date.

Neligan, Rev. William H. *Saintly Characters Recently Presented for Canonization.* P. J. Kenedy & Sons. New York. 1958.

Pietro Della Madre Di Dio, O.C.D. *Anita Cantieri.* Postulazione Dei Carmelitani Scalzi. Capannori-Lucca, Italy. 1955.

Purcell, Mary. *Matt Talbot and His Times.* Franciscan Herald Press. Chicago, Illinois. 1977.

Rachelina Ambrosini: Una Ragazza Vissuta per il Cielo. Fondazione Rachelina Ambrosini. Venticano, Italy. No date.

Rachelina Ambrosini, La Serva di Dio, Il Giglio d'Irpinia. Per la chiusura del "processo Diocesano." Benevento, Italy. 1995.

Rachelina Ambrosini: A Girl Who Lived for Heaven. Foundation Rachelina Ambrosini. Venticano, Italy. No date.

Rengers, Fr. Christopher, O.F.M.Cap. *The 33 Doctors of the Church.* TAN Books and Publishers, Inc. Rockford, Illinois. 2000.

Risso, Paolo. *Silvio Dissegna, Un Ragazzo Meraviglioso.* Editrice Elledici. Turin, Italy. 2002.

Rossi, C.M., Amedeo. *Antonietta Meo (Nennolina) Studio Biografico.* Tip. Le. Company. Piacenza, Italy. 1986.

Salaverri, Jose Maria. *Tal vez me hable Dios.* Ediciones S. M. Madrid, Spain. 1986.

———*Maybe God Will Speak to Me: The Story of Faustino Perez-Manglano.* Valencia, Spain. 1993.

———*The Four Yeses of Faustino.* Paper.

Setti, Mons. Giancarlo. *In the Light of the Epiphany: Maria Cristina Ogier.* Basilica di San Lorenzo. Firenze, Italy. 1977.

Silvestrelli, P. Stefano Igino. *Brigante No! Profilo Biografico di Maggiorino Vigolungo, Venerabile.* Edizioni Casa Di

Nazareth. Roma, Italy. 1988.

Teresa of Avila, Saint. *The Autobiography of St. Teresa of Avila: The Life of St. Teresa of Jesus.* David Lewis, trans.; Benedict Zimmerman, ed. Benziger, 1916; rpt. TAN Books and Publishers, Inc. Rockford, Illinois. 1997.

Un Santo in Carrozzella, Lettere del Servo di Dio Luigi Rocchi. Comitato per la Causa di Beatificazione di Luigi Rocchi. Tolentino, Italy. 1995.

Valabek, O.Carm., Redemptus Maria. *Profiles in Holiness I.* Edizioni Carmelitane. Rome, Italy. 1996.

———*Profiles in Holiness II.* Edizioni Carmelitane. Rome, Italy. 1999.

———*Profiles in Holiness III.* Edizioni Carmelitane. Rome, Italy. 2002.

Vanzan, Piersandro. *Antonietta Meo piccola evangelista della sofferenza.* Nuova Responsabilita. Febbraio. 2000.

Vatican Information Service. vis-news-en.blogspot.com

Verd-Conradi, S.J., Gabriel M. *Mari Carmen Gonzalez-Valerio: A Girl on Her Way to the Altars.* Madres Carmelitas Descalzas. Madrid, Spain. 1993.

Weiser, S.J., Francis X. *Kateri Tekakwitha.* The Kateri Center. Caughnawaga, P.Q., Canada. 1972.